# Outsmarting HPV

"A Quantum Medicine Perspective and Silver Solution to the Human Papilloma Virus (HPV) — A Modern Day Plague"

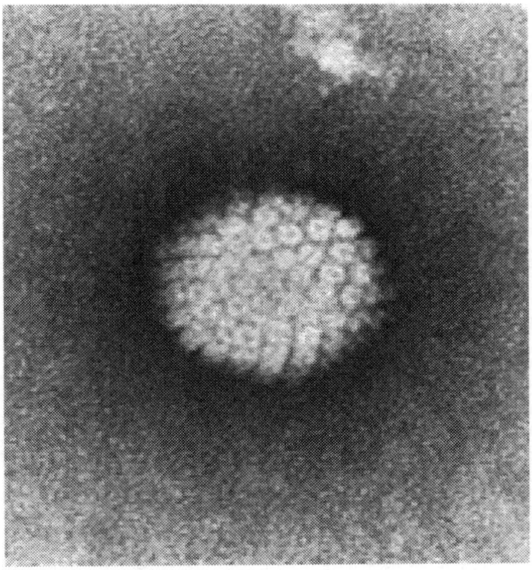

A Journey of Science and Discovery to Holism

By: Dr. Jay P. Vanden Heuvel Ph.D., I.M.D.

This book is dedicated to my father Richard for his fortitude and willingness to try a holistic approach when faced with no other options. Also to my wife Tracy who without her patience and belief in me, I would have went insane with frustration the last 20 years of my life.

I also want to thank my editor: Melanie Siebold for her diligence in research verifications.

# TABLE OF CONTENTS:

## Forward:
# A Modern Day Plague

The Human Papilloma virus (HPV) is a modern day plague with no pharmaceutical cure.

In this book, Dr. Jay describes the science and journey to a natural solution to HPV. He expertly teaches how women can help prevent and destroy HPV. Hopefully, women everywhere will celebrate as they learn the secret to helping the body heal itself with current and advanced pH balanced silver solution gels.

Dr. Jay reveals how the human body can be more successful at "healing" rather than just relying on the use of controversial vaccinations or pharmaceutical drug options alone. He documents the power of an all-natural silver gel and its anti-viral effects against human papilloma virus. Scientific studies help document that when silver stays in contact with bacteria, viruses, and yeast for 6 minutes, all three can be destroyed including the ubiquitous HPV.

Today approximately 96% of all women 18 years of age and older have been infected with the Human Papilloma virus significantly increasing the risk of vaginal infections, infertility and birth defects.

This little talked about approach helps reveal the scientific proof that will help change women's lives, because they can prevent and destroy the virus using all natural silver supplement gel along with powerful quantum aspects. This book helps prove that the body will heal itself if you give it the proper tools.

Experience a breath of fresh and balanced thinking from Dr. Jay as you read this terrific description of the way natural silver solutions destroy the previously incurable Human Papilloma virus. If you're looking for a brilliant new way to help the body integrate natural silver in conjunction with immune function to help prevent, protect, and destroy the human papilloma virus, this is it!

Dr. Jay expertly describes the science behind current and advanced silver sol gels. He reveals his research which gives women everywhere confidence and a sense of safety with an all-natural protocol to deal with vaginal infections that drugs cannot cure. As a naturopathic doctor I endorse this protocol, recommend this book, and congratulate him on his revolutionary findings. Women everywhere will celebrate their independence and control of vaginal viral infections.

This is a simple but comprehensive protocol against the dangerous Human Papilloma Virus. All the benefits outlined, documented, and witnessed here, are exceptional and women will rave with the independence it gives them to control their own vaginal wellness.

Every woman should read this book and make it part of their vaginal health protocols. Yes, every woman should be aware and active in the use of this type of protocol. I congratulate him on these exciting findings and a well written/researched book.

Gordon Pedersen Ph.D., N.D.

Board Certified in Anti-aging and Regenerative Medicine.

# PREFACE: All things Happen for a Reason…

My father was diagnosed with abdominal mesothelioma of the peritoneum in 1990. This is a cancer which is connected to an environmental toxin from plastics or asbestos. It is usually confined to the lungs. My father's mesothelioma was present throughout his peritoneum, which is part of the layers of the abdomen. He worked with plastics for 10 years in a manufacturing facility in Wisconsin.

A recorded surgical VHS video tape at the time showed cancer tissue (similar to a spider's web) throughout the abdomen and around the Liver. This video was a recording of the Laparoscopic examination. It also showed tissue samples being excised (biopsy). Then tissues were sent to a pathology lab for clinical diagnosis. A month later, a local oncologist and three nonlocal oncologists (Mayo clinic), all concurred with the diagnosis of Mesothelioma. He was told that there were no known successful allopathic treatments or cure available. Surgery was out of the question due to invasiveness. Chemotherapy would only make him sick and basically ineffective. Radiation treatment also was invaluable with this type of cancer. His voiced prognosis from the local oncologist was "You have maybe six months to live. So, get your affairs in order. Go fishing".

Being of a medical background, with studies in nursing and an associate's degree in surgical technology, the family asked for help in what all these big words, diagnosis, and prognosis meant. "Go fishing" pretty much summed it up. Even though there was no expiration date on the bottom of his feet (sarcasm is a coping mechanism). My father expressed he wasn't ready to die at 58 years of age. He wanted to live.

In 1990, I was studying and using standardized proanthocyanidins (a powerful "vitamin C" type antioxidant) from Maritime pine bark out of France. These phytochemicals are also found in grape seeds. Since chemotherapy, radiation, or surgery, were not even an option, proanthocyanidins presented "something".

I was also experimenting with an herbal brew of four herbs commonly found in Wisconsin for Dad. The herbal concoction came from the historical Ojibwe Indian pharmacopeia. Today it is commonly known as "Essiac Tea" or "E-Tea". This ancient herbal brew was made famous by a Canadian Nurse named Renee Caisse. The word "Essiac" was a code name for this brew that Renee invented herself (she spelt her name Caisse backwards). She used many different names for this historical blend in her career due to some persecution hassles while living in Canada. She had used E-Tea with great success with terminally ill cancer patients and the powers that be, didn't like it (she actually spent many months -more than once - in jail for doing so). The Canadian Parliament heavily frowned upon this type of unsubstantiated therapy. She was considered "practicing medicine without a license". Even though she was working with terminally ill cancer patients the medical system had given up on. It is worth noting that Essiac tea was endorsed and tested in the United States by President Kennedy's personal physician, Dr. Charles A. Brusch.

I learned to boil down the four herbs of Sheep Sorrel, Burdock, Slippery Elm bark, and Turkish Rhubarb root, with water for 24 hours into a mash. Steeping it and straining it, turning the mash once over every two hours of the 24 hours. Then bottle it into sterile amber containers for my father to drink as a tea. It is historically known as a blood purifier and powerful Liver detoxifier. At least again, we felt we were doing something. Two years had elapsed since the diagnosis, but my father didn't.

In 1992 I began reading a book called "Sharks Don't Get Cancer" by Dr. I. William Lane and Linda Comac. The premise was these creatures (Sharks) don't have any bones, only cartilage. Sharks are comprised of mostly cartilage, which is flexible soft tissue, like what is in your ears and nose. What was postulated and presented throughout this book was that cartilage contained something called anti-angiogenesis factor. Genesis means to form or create, angio refers to blood vessel, and anti- simply means to go against or stop. If you read the word right to left, anti-angiogenesis means "to stop blood vessel growth". The idea was that this substance could help stop excessive blood vessel growth, which is what cancer cells use in high supply. It has been noted that cancer cells can grow roughly 20 times faster than normal healthy cells, so they tend to need a larger blood vessel supply. In theory if you consume shark cartilage, you are providing higher amounts of anti-angiogenesis factor. This may starve out the cancer cells (hence the title of the book). However, it has been proven about a decade later (in Great White sharks) that this may not be true. But in 1992, it was all we had to go on then. Again, we decided to do something versus nothing. After all, the medical advice was to "go fishing" (so we literally were).

"Here Dad, eat this pine bark, drink these weeds, and have some ground up shark". I often said to him jokingly. Humor was also an important factor to healing (he had made it two years now). His faith was strong and he felt he wasn't ready to die. It was an initiation to the hidden world of natural health. We didn't know it, but we were using a holistic and quantum approach. Holistic meant we were treating a whole host of mind, body, and spiritual practices. Things like humor, herbs, diet, exercise, prayer, etc. A Quantum approach meant we were using our creativity to help find new ideas or solutions. We found "aha" moments regarding his healing. The proof was him still standing upright in front of me.

To everyone's amazement who knew him, in 1996 my father was still thriving (obviously, the expiration date the allopath's gave him was incorrect). He had pain, abdominal distention, and daily struggles, but he was still very much alive. His local oncologist on subsequent visits even went so far as to refuse or even acknowledge his survival. He sarcastically stated at one appointment "What are you doing alive?" as he scribed (I know this because I was there). The Doctor also assured him "You know this will eventually kill you". His advice was to prescribe morphine and eventual hospice care if needed. My Dad just shook his head. He couldn't believe this oncologist wasn't the least bit interested in what he was taking.

Soon after all that, I was visiting my parents one day when irony paid a visit. Irony visited in the form of a phone call. I just happened to pick up the ringing phone (back when phones were attached to a wall).

It was a call from the Canadian Mesothelioma Society. They asked to speak to my father, Richard. They called him that day because he was (in 1996) one of the oldest living survivors of Mesothelioma they knew of in the world. The conversation went like this: "Hello. Yes, this is Richard". Then I heard him say, "No, I am not seeing a doctor. The doctors can't help me anyway. No, I am not doing chemotherapy". After a long pause he continued, "My son is helping me. He has me taking some weeds that grow in a ditch, some kind of pine tree, and ground up shark bones". He then hung up after a couple minutes, disgusted. He then turned to me and said "They don't really want to know how I am doing this, just what doctor, chemo, or radiation, I am using". He was so upset. So was I.

Why didn't they want to know what he was doing? Why were they not the least bit interested in how he was doing this? As you already guessed, it wasn't allopathic scientifically proven patented medicine. That is not a slam by the way. It is just baffling that he may have helped show an adjunct to consider and that his natural treatment wouldn't even be considered.

Time marched on, no further calls, no further doctor requests. We continued the protocol adding fiber, liver purifiers, diet modifications, and even some hydrogen peroxide.

My father did eventually pass away in 2002. It was a twelve year struggle versus the six months given. But his story (and my journey) was not to end there. His death certificate showed the cause of death was Emphysema. That demise was because cigarettes were a lifelong habit he enjoyed since adolescence and could not give up from his lifestyle.

As we know, there is no cure for death. Emphysema contributed to this death. But his eventual exit wasn't from the death sentence he received in 1990. He got 12 years extra (he and my family would agree) from using holistic, quantum approaches, and faith in a higher power. We learned a valuable lesson that consciousness does matter.

Last, but not least, our family convinced our mother to do an autopsy on him. We were inquisitive as to what happened to the cancer? The autopsy revealed no cancer, just emphysema. There wasn't any evidence left of the original mesothelioma diagnosis at all. The Mayo clinic was sent a copy of the autopsy in 2002 for comment. They notified our family that the diagnosis (mesothelioma) must have been misdiagnosed.

Misdiagnosed? Seriously it is baffling how a video tape, biopsy, pathological report, and four oncologists confirming Mesothelioma in 1990, was now so easily dismissed. Couldn't they acknowledge a reversal? How about spontaneous remission? They could only conclude the diagnosis must have been wrong to begin with? Would that establishment have reversed this diagnosis if allopathic treatment methods alleviated his condition? Common sense says no.

All things do happen for a reason. My father's diagnosis, willingness to try new things, valor, and eventually the end result, were instrumental in my own journey to become integrated. Along this time frame, many people in my home area started asking me for this type of help, just by word of mouth. I knew what we did was not a "cure all" for anyone, but it sure was an eye opener. Modern medicine is not always so modern I thought. I had to know more. These types of natural methods were never even mentioned ever in any of my initial medical trainings.

I went onto become an American Board Certified Reflexologist. I practiced and taught Reflexology for 10 years. I also went on to become a Certified Flower Therapist. I completed a Bachelor's and Masters of Science degree in Natural Health too. In September of 2002, I received a board certification as a Holistic Health Practitioner (AADP). Then graduated as a Ph.D. in 2003 in Holistic Health (England). In 2011, I received my second Ph.D. in Traditional Naturopathy (Alabama). In April 2015, I received a Doctorate and Ph.D. in Integrative Medicine from Quantum University in Hawaii with an emphasis on quantum physics. I became Board Certified as a Doctor of Integrative Medicine (BOIM) and Board Certified as a Doctor of Humanitarian Medicine in the World Organization of Natural Medicine (WONM).

I've been blessed with the humbling privilege of seeing over 17,000 customers so far in my career. I have been able to lecture around the world, done talk radio, television, written numerous articles, a book, published DVD's, CD's, and am humbled by natural healing methods every day.

So, all things do happen for a reason. Helping my father by integrative methods with a terminal diagnosis, using nature (sometimes as a last resort, although it should be a first), you can witness a miracle. You can witness "aha" moments.

These "aha" moments present themselves daily now. I have come to realize you need to open your mind and look elsewhere for options. We all have experienced somewhere in our lives, that what we consider traditional medicine, sometimes fails to bring about a positive outcome. Like in my father's case we had to look elsewhere. We had to integrate with or without a traditional doctors blessing. Hence, I have become very passionate about (and practice) quantum medicine. Quantum medicine in my opinion is the medicine of the future.

In conclusion, all attempts at healing require new waves of possibility and of course, to never give up. In this preface, my father needed a quantum "leap" in healing to live on twelve years. I also needed a quantum "leap" of creativity to go from allopathic thinking, to integration of holistic and vibrational approaches. The fact remains there is a time and place for prescriptions and surgical procedures, true. But this experience more than motivated me to become integrative.

This book continues to explore and help prove Holistic and Quantum approaches do work! The following is a proven protocol concept originally developed from a published thesis, outsmarting a disease that modern medicine really does not have a solid answer for, the Human Papilloma Virus.

Dr. Jay P. Vanden Heuvel Ph.D., IMD

# INTRODUCTION: CANCER, A QUANTUM VIEW

According to the CDC (Center of Disease Control) history of diseases, in 1900 cancer was ranked #8 in top ten causes of death. Today cancer is #2 (1). Elimination of some infectious diseases has helped changed many of the top ten rankings over the last century, but these eliminations did little to halt cancer climbing to become #2. We know now stress and the environment are the biggest contributors to cancer and infectious diseases which still run rampant. Infections, like HPV, play a pivotal role in its climb.

All Cancer prognoses are generally gaged in what is known as cancer survival rate. A time period that is currently a five year survival rate. According to the National Cancer Institute (www.cancer.gov), this five-year survival rate is the time period traditionally associated with a good prognosis. Adopted around 1950, it helped make cancer statistics look better and gave an impression that we, as a medical society, were "winning the war on cancer". It was a reductionist way of thinking. Just assigning a cancer survival rate is not a realistic way of "winning". It has been shown in the year 2000 by the American Medical Association, that this has had little relationship to changes in the mortality of cancer (2).

The focus does need to be on mortality, detection, treatment advancements, and prevention. But the war on cancer is far from over. A different approach is needed to stop "fighting" cancer. A new focus (a paradigm shift or new wave of possibility) should be directed at the cause. My father's diagnosis, simply, was environmentally influenced (asbestos). An occupational hazard from the foundry he worked for.

For example, an article in Science magazine Jan. 2015 entitled Bad Luck and Cancer, argued that most cancers are out of our control. In went on to say that researchers report the majority of cancer types, are the result of pure chance. That most of these cancers are the result of random genetic mutations. That statement may be true but not conclusive. Asbestos exposure or HPV infections are not always random! In the case of HPV infection causing cervical cancer (not random), understanding cancer in general we become better equipped at dealing with it. The article failed to mention "influence" on random mutations of genes. It was more geared to help us feel like "Cancer is not our fault". The article is not direct, the complacency is. So in this book we will explore a more in depth understanding of why mutations happen at all. Using something called epigenetics (influence), and also a concept of biological terrain, and of course knowing this helps with the greatest treatment of all - prevention. A more detailed quantum view of cancer in general is also needed here. We as a medical science have a long way to go to deter this potential number one killer called cancer (it is poised to edge out heart disease for the #1 spot in America, in just a few years).

A good place to start and a good mantra I once heard Dr. Mark Hyman mention in public was: there is "I" in illness, but "we" in wellness. How true. Quantum physics does teach us that Consciousness is the ground of all being. And that consciousness creates possibilities. "We" should all be a part of the solution. "We" all need to work from an integrative perspective for anyone's health. It helps construct a positive entanglement (tangled hierarchy) for the common good of all involved.

Integration in medicine, with a more holistic/quantum approach, can help win this so called war. This is the medicine of the future, quantum. It can help find solutions to our many human ills that modern medicine may fail to find. By being creative and breaking out of paradigms that blind us to natural possibilities. Many agree modern medicine would be much better served if it would change its current paradigms. Hopefully, modern allopathic medicine will try to embrace that soon versus patented medicine only designed by capitalistic monopolies.

Medical science in the last century turned a blind eye to the power of healing by holistic approaches, in favor of capitalism. Patented medicine is big money. Just watch a few documentaries like "Bought". For the love of God, just because we can't patent Broccoli, doesn't mean we shouldn't continue to explore it deeper for its unlocked health potentials as medicine. "We" as a society can help change the paradigm of today's science if only we demand to integrate nature as the ultimate healer. Nature is multi-dimensional and energetic in its own right. Did you know around 70% of all pharmaceuticals were discovered from a plant to begin with?

An "aha" moment I have had in my last 24 years, is that Cancer is not a disease, but a symptom. It is also not always a death sentence. Its outcome does depend very much on the location of it, the speed of it, and early detection of it. But working to eliminate the cause is most likely what Richard Nixon meant when he as president, declared a "war on Cancer".

Cancer does result from the development of abnormal properties in normal cells from factors which we can't always identify, but suspect. This contributes to normal cells dividing excessively and spreading to other locations. This is an abnormal development. It can be caused by mutations in a cell DNA that occur from factors such as chemicals, radiation, ultraviolet light, and chromosome replication errors. These factors are known as mutagens. Are they random? Not if we know how to avoid them. Yet, they do alter DNA by changing nucleotide bases. These mutagens can even change the shape of DNA. The altered DNA produces errors in replication and protein synthesis. Our bodies start making bad copies. These mutagens influence cell growth and cell division for sure, but also contribute to cellular aging in general.

Viruses are also a known mutagen. They too have the ability to cause cancer by altering cell genes. Viruses change cells by combining their genetic material with the host cell's DNA. The infected cell is then regulated by the new combined viral genes. It now has the ability to undergo abnormal growth.

Several viruses have been linked to certain types of cancer in humans. The Epstein-Barr virus has been linked to Burkitt's lymphoma, the hepatitis B virus has been linked to liver cancer, and the human papilloma viruses (HPV) have been linked to cervical cancer (3).

Using quantum creativity (thinking quantum, be creative) let's explore the possibility of a non-invasive quantum approach to outsmarting HPV. Quantum creativity enables us to solve unusual problems. This book is that, a manifested solution from a possibility, into a proven reproducible protocol.

Throughout this book, we explore holistic methodology (i.e. biological terrain management, pH balancing, diet/nutrition, detoxification etc.) and quantum approaches (vibrational frequency of pathogens vs. vibrational remedies, chakra balancing, energy medicine, etc.) along with using aqua sol-silver technology/frequency to greatly reduce this risk and practice prevention.

Much of the research here includes several decades of reputable lab study/ research by such University's as Brigham Young (BYU), and Penn State University, as well as credentialed authorities. Along with, my own private practice (in clinic for 20 years) using a protocol method utilizing something called Silver sol gel, along with flower therapy, supplements, and understanding epigenetics, just to name a few.

This book concludes with actual clinical case studies of clients with abnormal pap smears, which have been verified as corrected by follow up Pap tests, by using a quantum and holistic approach. I can only hope this quantum/holistic protocol approach with silver technology and vibrational medicine will become a mainstream complimentary and integrative approach of HPV prevention worldwide.

There is no cure for HPV infection allopathically at this time.

You will also see there were 18 women who volunteered to use a Quantum Holistic approach using Silver Aqua Sol Gel technology in the complimentary care of abnormal Pap tests and positive HPV testing. They all volunteered to use this silver sol gel protocol and were followed up by their respective regular physicians as well. They were diagnosed with varying degrees of abnormal pap smears tests (indicating cervical tissue dysplasia and cancer) and all had tested positive for HPV.

The case studies were conducted over the course of four years (2010-2014). It took this length of time to find the 18 volunteers. They all agreed and expressed verbal consent to use this approach. They were determined to be candidates for the silver sol gel protocol based on a positive test for HPV.

All 18, using the quantum holistic approach and silver sol gel protocol, cleared their abnormal pap smears within six months. Some volunteers were advised to wait longer for a follow up Pap test by their follow up physicians, which was dependent on age. Most chose to test sooner even though the cost of follow up testing was out of pocket to determine efficacy. This was encouraged as well, to help with more immediate results of the protocol.

All 18 women are considered within normal limits (negative, stage 0 on repeat Pap, or reported as no cellular abnormalities) by their respective medical personnel. They were deemed to be HPV free going forward. Only one of them had a history of HPV vaccination prior to diagnosis.

# Chapter 1:
# HUMAN PAPILLOMA VIRUS (HPV) AND DETECTION

According to the Merck Manual (Nineteenth edition) there are roughly 40 - 50 types of Human papillomavirus (HPV) typically transmitted thru sexual contact. HPV infection is a cause of nearly all cervical cancer in women and most cervical abnormalities (4).

Currently, a Papanicolaou (Pap) test or liquid-based cytology is used to detect abnormal cells that may develop into cancer of the cervix. The cervix, a neck like structure of the uterus, is located at the top of the vagina canal. This type of screening test is designed to help find early signs of cancer that may develop in the future or is already developing. It is not necessarily designed to diagnose cancer or HPV infection.

HPV testing is done in conjunction with a Pap test. An HPV test is generally done on cells that are removed at the same time as a Pap smear. HPV testing is usually done for women over the age of 30. (This is because younger women tend to clear the virus from their body more readily and have fewer consequences from it.)

The testing is done with a speculum inserted into the vagina for entry and visualization. A small sample of cells are taken from the cervix area and placed on a glass slide. The slide is sent to pathology for examination and diagnosis. If abnormal cells are found, further Pap tests are performed at a later time, especially if low grade changes are noted.

If abnormal cells persist, women are usually then assessed with a colposcopy. During a colposcopy inspection, invasive biopsies can be taken and abnormal areas can be removed with a simple procedure, typically with a cauterizing loop or by freezing (cryotherapy). Other treatments, which are also invasive minor operations, include Laser treatment or a Cone Biopsy. Many of these abnormal Pap tests can result from an infection of HPV.

The United States Preventative Services Task Force (USPSTF) recommends screening for cervical cancer with a Pap smear every three years for women ages 21 to 65. More recently as of July 21, 2014 the USPSTF advises those that want less screening, women ages 30 to 65, can choose to undergo a combination of Pap smear and HPV test every five years instead. These current allopathic techniques carry some risk and some like biopsy or cryo-surgery, are extremely invasive. There is also a high probability of reoccurrence of HPV, since the virus itself is so small. There is also a possibility of reinfection.

Currently, allopathic measures have no definitive answer to eliminating HPV. Preventative measures such as condoms, which are strongly encouraged, also show no definitive proof of prevention from this type of infection. Detection with Pap smears has been able to reduce the incidence and fatalities of cervical cancer in the developed world. Still there were 11,000 cases and 3,900 deaths just in the U.S. in 2008 (5).

HPV is estimated to be the most common sexually transmitted infection in the United States. According to the Center of Disease Control in 2014, fifty percent of all sexually active people will have an HPV infection in their lifetime.

According to www.worldlifeexpectancy.com in 2014; the United States ranking for death from cervical cancer (all ages of female) is ranked 34th. It is ranked as high as 15th for females within 25-34 years of age. Cervical cancer also has substantial mortality rates in resource-poor areas; worldwide. The African country of Guinea for example, has a death rate for females of 23.7 per 100,000 people. It is the highest in the world. There are an estimated 490,000 cases and 270,000 deaths each year worldwide attributed to HPV/Cervical Cancer.

HPV infection is definitely the most frequently sexually transmitted disease (STD) in the world. Current methods of prevention include abstinence, condoms, vaccination schedules, and microbicides. There are tests for certain types of HPV as well. Most of the time HPV testing is not done because it is assumed that HPV will clear out on its own, naturally.

Current prevention methods are not stemming the fact that HPV is (by most estimates), to be the most common sexually transmitted infection in the United States as well. Most sexually active women (men too) will probably acquire genital HPV infection at some point in their life. The American

Social Health Association reports that about 75-80% of sexually active Americans will be infected with HPV at some point in their lifetime. By the age of 50, more than 80% of American women will have contracted at least one strain of genital HPV.

## Chapter 2:
# HPV DISCUSSION IN WOMENS HEALTH

***Women's Gynecological Concerns and HPV*** — It's estimated that one in four women suffer from some type of vaginal problem every day (6). Most of these issues can be resolved on their own with good hygiene, gynecological exams and treatment, or home health care. Some of these vaginal problems, especially HPV, can lead all the way to cancer. Many times, disease can manifest without any symptoms to warn women of an impending danger.

The most concerning of all vaginal problems is cervical cancer. This is the 3rd most common gynecologic cancer and 8th most common cancer among women in U.S. The known causative pathogen is the Human papillomavirus (7). Nobel laureate Harald zur Hausen is credited with discovering that HPV infection causes cervical cancer thirty years ago.

The vaginal cavity is a warm and moist area. It has its own specific pH (potential of Hydrogen) of < 4.5, making it an acidic environment. In pH chemistry terms, 7.0 pH is considered neutral. Anything above 7.0 is alkaline, anything below 7.0 is considered acidic. This specific pH is important to helping maintain a homeostatic balance to the area and deter infection.

So many factors will influence the outcome of an infection in the vaginal area. Examples can be poor hygiene, pH imbalance, hormone imbalance, energetic influence or frequency, introduction of foreign pathogens (HPV), even epigenetics. Let's consider for now just the HPV virus pathogen.

***Viral Background*** — A virus itself is considered a small (sub-microscopic) parasite, a type of opportunistic infection. They are found in air, water, and in all forms of macro-life. Viruses have a very notable 'cause of death and disease' throughout the world. For many viruses, such as influenza, Ebola, KPC-1, or the avian bird flu, there are virtually no beneficial drugs or treatment (8).

Viruses are not considered living organisms. A virus depends on living cells (bacterial, plant, or animal/human) to reproduce. Viruses, like HPV, have an outer cover of protein (sometimes lipid) and an RNA or DNA core of segments. This can also be considered in Quantum physics as an example of a "tangled hierarchy". A tangled hierarchy is a type of circular logic. Viruses bring this query to mind. What came first, the protein covering or the RNA/DNA segments? It is now known, it takes protein to make DNA and it takes DNA to make protein. Let that sink in. It puzzles many how and why viruses even exist!

Infection with HPV occurs when the HPV virus attaches itself to host (living) cells. These cells are usually in the cervix area in the vaginal canal. The viral RNA or DNA segments from the virus then enter host cells to begin a replication of viral genetic instructions. RNA segments replicate in the cytoplasm of a host cell and DNA segments in the nucleus. The host cell typically ruptures and dies. It then releases copies of the original virus to other surrounding host cells. This continues a cycle of infection. Left untreated, this can inflict terrible damage on the human body. In the case of HPV infection the result is cervical cancer. Ultimately if the HPV cannot attach itself to a healthy cell in the first place, it wouldn't even have the ability to inject damaged segments at all. This would result in no infection or cervical cancer in the first place. Silver sol technology, explored later, provides a preventative measure to this line of defense reasoning ('mechanisms of action' Chap. 6).

Royal Raymond Rife was a scientist who passed away in 1971. He helped develop technology and many inventions in his day. One of them was the first virus microscope in 1920. By 1933, he perfected what was known as the Universal Microscope or Rife microscope. It was capable of 60,000 time magnification of normal size. He is attributed as the first human to see an active virus. He noted viruses change form, to accommodate changes in their environment. That they also change in response to carcinogens and can transform normal cells in tumor cells. He also noted a virus has a "specific frequency". Frequency will be discussed also in more detail later. Today we know viruses cause many diseases that we simply don't have pharmaceutical drugs to cure. Sometimes physicians prescribe an antibiotic in the case of viral infection, which is ineffective on a virus.

***HPV Types*** — Let's continue the breakdown of HPV infection even further. Human papillomavirus (HPV) is a DNA virus from the papillomavirus family that is capable of infecting all humans. Like all papillomaviruses,

HPVs establish productive infections only in keratinocytes of the skin or mucous membranes. Most HPV infections are subclinical and will cause no physical symptoms; however, in some people subclinical infections will become clinical and may cause benign papilloma's (such as warts [verrucae] or squamous cell papilloma), or cancers of the cervix, uterus, vulva, vagina, penis, oropharynx and anus (4).

Over 120 HPV types have been identified and are referred to by a number. As previously stated, up to 50 types of HPV are typically transmitted through sexual contact and infect the ano-genital region.

Specific HPV numbered types (16 and 18) can even cause infections of a unique type of oropharyngeal (throat) cancer. For example, a very famous actor, contracted HPV throat cancer from the strains HPV 16 and HPV 18 supposedly from oral sex, which made all the mainstream media outlets. In fact, head and neck cancers associated with HPV are on the rise. According to an article in the Scientific American March 2015, "Cancer Goes Viral", Ohio State University medical oncologist Maura Gillison, has studied men with oropharyngeal cancer for three decades. She found from 1984 to 1989 sixteen percent of oropharyngeal cancers tested positive for HPV. By 2005 that figure skyrocketed to 73 percent. These figures are shifting the burden of HPV from women to men. No data currently exists to prove vaccines protect against HPV-positive oropharyngeal cancer.

Again noted in the Merck manual, HPV is known to cause skin warts (verrucae); genital warts; and cervical cancer/carcinoma. It is universal, very common, and often recurrent. Less common is anal carcinoma and head/neck carcinoma.

Current allopathic therapy for abnormal cells of the cervix in women includes cryotherapy; surgical resection; radiation therapy plus chemotherapy; interferon (genital); podophyllin (genital); and imiquimod. Prevention of HPV is allopathically (Merck) noted as vaccines (4 sub types of HPV) and condoms.

***HPV Screening*** — The 2012 American Cancer Society and ASCCP (American Society for Colposcopy and Cervical Pathology) Screening Guidelines recommend continued close surveillance of women who are positive for high-risk HPV strains, which are the HPV subtypes that can cause cancer (HR-HPV), in particular cervical, vaginal, and vulvar cancers of the female genital tract. These recommendations are regardless of whether the

Pap test is negative. The new guidelines specifically address situations of negative Pap smears with +HR-HPV. The guidelines now include subtyping for HPV strains 16 and 18, which are known to cause approximately 70% of cervical cancers, with the other oncogenic strains responsible for the rest. It has been found that women with HPV 16 and 18 and a negative Pap have a greater than 10% risk of CIN 3+ (the immediate precursor to invasive cervical cancer) within 5 years of testing positive. The risk of development of pre-cancer for the other high-risk HPV subtypes is lower.

The options for following a patient with a negative Pap and +HR-HPV:

1) Follow up in one year with a Pap and HPV co-testing, and if either the Pap is abnormal or the HPV is still positive, then the patient should undergo a colposcopy of the cervix.

2) Immediate HPV subtyping and referral to colposcopy for +HPV 16/18.

3) Immediate HPV subtyping and if the HR-HPV is non-HPV 16/18, then repeat Pap and HPV co-testing in one year. If in one year either the Pap is abnormal or the HPV is still positive, then a colposcopy should be performed (9).

***HPV Symptoms and Prognosis*** — Human papillomavirus infection can cause a squamous cell carcinoma of the cervix. Cervical neoplasia is asymptomatic. The first symptom of early cervical cancer if presented is usually irregular, often post-coital vaginal bleeding. Again, diagnosis is accomplished through a screening of the cervix (Pap test) and biopsy. Staging of these findings is clinical.

Cervical cancer results from cervical intraepithelial neoplasia (CIN), which appears to be caused by infection with HPV number types 16, 18,31,33,35, or 39. The risk factors include: being of younger age at their first intercourse, having a high number of sexual partners, and men whose previous partners had cervical cancer. Also cigarette smoking and immunodeficiency are cofactors. CIN is usually evident on a Pap test and is graded as 1 (mild cervical dysplasia), 2 (moderate dysplasia), 3 (severe dysplasia and carcinoma in situ), 4 (it has spread to adjacent organs or distant organs). Clinical staging of cervical carcinoma involves tissue depths for a larger database of study ranging from 0-4B.

Studies have shown that infections with multiple types of HPV do occur.

This tends to increase the severity of cervical disease (10). About 80 -85% of all cervical cancers are squamous cell carcinoma, the rest adenocarcinomas. Sarcomas and small cell neuroendocrine tumors are rare. Invasive cervical cancer usually spreads by direct extension into surrounding tissues or via the lymphatic's to the pelvic lymph nodes. Hematagenous spread of the cancer is possible.

Left untreated, the prognosis (squamous cell carcinoma) is based on 5 year survival rates. Stage 1 is 80-90%. Stage 2 is 60-75%. Stage 3 is 30-40%. Stage 4 is 0-15%.

A subset to HPV infection is other vaginal conditions often noted for clinical evaluation. Well up to 50% of all OB/GYN visits are for pelvic pain/discomfort (pain/itching) and discharge. Current Allopathic treatment usually includes Antibiotics mostly, with follow up for these subsets. A tradeoff then exists with substantial use of antibiotics, known as a vaginal yeast infection or candida. Antibiotics are of no value in HPV treatment (since it is a virus) but may be prescribed for the subsets.

# Chapter 3:
# THE VACCINE DEBATE

***What we know (so far)*** — A common way to build immunity against a viral attack is by vaccination. It is the known allopathic medicine of today and is considered the standard of building (herd) immunity. In the case of HPV, it is considered the frontline of HPV prevention.

Vaccines historically are similar to the principle of homeopathy. It started out with the idea of introducing small pieces of an antigen or attenuated (dead or weakened germ) tissues in a medium. This helps prepare the body to encode a defense against an invader or pathogen by building immune cells precisely against it. In ancient China around 200 B.C. they first used powdered scabs as a vaccine. Basically, the body can practice fighting the disease by making antibodies from vaccinations.

It is worth noting that modern vaccines are known to have risks. Each individual may react differently once a vaccine has passed the first line of defense; the skin. The biggest risk recognized is that a small amount of individuals may contract the very disease they are being vaccinated against. Outcomes can be hard to predict.

Some debate centers around questionable ingredients or preservatives in any vaccine serum as well. But let's keep the focus solely on HPV vaccines efficacy.

Let's compare what we know of HPV vaccines from multiple sources (11, 12). HPV vaccines are newly developed vaccines. There are currently two HPV vaccines on the market.

The first is Gardasil, which was licensed by the U.S. Food and Drug Administration (FDA) in 2006. It is the one recommended for females between the ages of 9-26. The second HPV vaccine named Cervarix was licensed in 2009. The Center for Disease Control's (CDC) Advisory Committee on Immunization Practices recommended HPV vaccine for males between ages of 11-21 as of October 2011.

The vaccines aim to prevent cervical cancer, but in no way do they treat it. For the vaccine dosage, 3 doses are given intramuscular (1st month, followed by 2nd month, finally 6th month). Each vaccine is effective only if you get all three doses. Only 57.3% of adolescent girls and 34.6% of adolescent boys get even one dose (13). The vaccines are recommended before sexual activity even begins. It is not recommended after age 26 for females and age 21 for males.

***The Controversy*** — Controversy ensues over whether or not vaccines for HPV are safe and effective.

According to a published article in the Journal of the American Medical Association (JAMA) August, 19th 2009 entitled "Post licensure of Safety Surveillance for Quadrivalent Human Papillomavirue Recombinant Vaccine", the study looked at patterns for all adverse events reported to the Vaccine Adverse Event Reporting System (VAERS). From June 2006 through December 32, 2008 (it did not include Cervarix), the findings were not that much different from other vaccines recommended and studied. The Food and Drug Administration (FDA) and Center for Disease Control (CDC) concluded that the HPV vaccine continues to be safe and effective. They also concluded that the benefits continue to outweigh its risks. They stated it is a reason for reduction in HPV infection.

The JAMA study's main findings showed more than 23 million doses were administered nationally since June of 2006. A total of 12,424 reports to VAERS were of adverse events following HPV vaccination through December of 2008. Some common effects or events included Syncope, local reaction at injection site, dizziness, nausea, and headache.

Of the 12,424 reports (VAERS), 772 adverse events (6%) were described as "serious". An adverse event is considered serious if it is life threatening, may cause death, permanent disability, hospitalization, or abnormal conditions at birth. The report showed that there were 32 deaths and 2 reports of unusual neurological illness specifically from the "serious" events. The report did question the 32 deaths and that they could be explained by factors outside of the vaccine. There was an increase reported with syncope and pulmonary emboli. They compared this to what has been found in other vaccines for the same age and gender. They admitted these findings needed further investigation.

Later in 2013, significant discrepancies were uncovered by Sharlene Bidini, RD, CSO. In a new HPV vaccine effectiveness study published in the Journal of Infectious Diseases (14). It evaluated data from the National Health and Nutrition Examination Surveys (NHANES), 2003-2006 and 2007-2010. Her conclusion was; reduction in HPV prevalence can NOT be claimed to be due to the effectiveness of HPV vaccinations. The data clearly shows that it was the unvaccinated girls in this group that had the best outcome.

She pointed out in this study that in 2007-2010, the overall prevalence of HPV infection was 50 percent in vaccinated girls (14-19 years), but only 38.6% in unvaccinated girls of the same age. So, the findings showed, HPV prevalence dropped 27.3% in the unvaccinated girls, but only declined by 5.8% in the vaccinated group. In four out of five different measures, the unvaccinated girls had a lower incidence of HPV.

The original JAMA study concluded that HPV vaccine effectiveness was high. But this new inspection and evidence pointed to a serious design flaw when compared to Bidini's work. Again, the unvaccinated group had a better outcome, evidenced by the JAMA's own study results.

***Safety of HPV Vaccines*** — What about HPV vaccine safety? Issues regarding safety continue today despite JAMA, FDA, CDC, and Licensed Manufacturer's for the vaccines, state clearly otherwise.

Consider a case where HPV DNA fragments were found in the blood of a teenage girl who died after receiving the Gardasil vaccine (all three doses). This was published in the peer reviewed J. Advances in Bioscience and Biotechnology (15). The girl was noted as being healthy. She died in her sleep six months after receiving her third and final dose. A full autopsy revealed no cause of death. Sin Hang Lee with the Milford Molecular Laboratory in Connecticut confirmed the presence of HPV-16 L1 gene DNA in the girl's postmortem blood and spleen tissue. These DNA fragments are a component in the HPV vaccine. The fragments are protected from degradation by binding firmly to an aluminum preservative used in the vaccine serum. Lee described "The significance of these HPV DNA fragments of a vaccine origin found in post-mortem materials is not clear and warrants further investigation".

Lee suggested the presence of HPV DNA fragments of vaccine could offer a plausible explanation for the high immunogenicity of Gardasil. This means that the vaccine has the ability to initiate an exaggerated immune response.

He did also point out that the rate of anaphylaxis in girls receiving Gardasil is higher than normal—reportedly 5 to 20 times higher than any other school-based vaccination program.

Could Gardasil actually increase the risk of cervical cancer? Judicial Watch information says yes. They claim it supposedly came straight from the licensed manufacturer to the FDA prior to the vaccines approval. Based on the licensed manufacturers own research, if you have been exposed to HPV strains 16 or 18 prior to receipt of Gardasil, women could increase their risk of precancerous lesions by 44.6%.

"The FDA adverse event reports on the HPV vaccine read like a catalog of horrors. Any state or local government now beset by (manufacturer) lobbying campaigns to mandate this HPV vaccine for young girls ought to take a look at these adverse health reports."

—Tom Fitton, President of Judicial Watch

As of May 13, 2013, VAERS had received 29,686 reports of adverse events following HPV vaccinations, including 136 reports of death, as well as 922 reports of disability, and 550 life-threatening adverse events.

The Judicial Watch announced it had received from FOIA (Freedom of Information Act) documents from the DHHS (Dept. of Health and Human Services), which showed that the National Vaccine Injury Compensation Program has awarded $5,877,710 to forty-nine victims for harm resulting from the HPV vaccine in March 20, 2013. This represents $120,000 per claim.

According to a press release: "On March 12, 2013, The Health Resources and Services Administration (HRSA), an agency of DHHS, provided Judicial Watch with documents revealing the following information:

49 of 200 claims filed have been compensated for injury or death caused from the (HPV) vaccine. Of the 49 compensated claims, 47 were for injury caused from the (HPV) vaccine. The additional 2 claims were for death caused due to the vaccine.

92 of the total 200 claims filed are still pending. Of those pending claims, 87 of the claims against the (HPV) vaccine were filed for injury. The remaining 5 claims were filed for death.

59 claims have been dismissed outright by VICP. The alleged victims were not compensated for their claims against the HPV vaccine. Of the claims dismissed, 57 were for injuries, 2 were for deaths allegedly caused by the HPV vaccine.

"This new information from the government shows that the serious safety concerns about the use of Gardasil have been well-founded," said Judicial Watch President Tom Fitton. He also stated "Public health officials should stop pushing Gardasil on children."

A systematic review of pre- and post-licensure trials of the HPV vaccine by researchers at University of British Columbia in 2013 entitled: Human papillomavirus (HPV) vaccines as an option for preventing cervical malignancies: (how) effective and safe? It published that the vaccine's effectiveness is not only overstated (through the use of selective reporting) but also unproven. In it they stated, "The claim that HPV vaccination will result in approximately 70% reduction of cervical cancers is made despite the fact that the clinical trials data have not demonstrated to date that the vaccines have actually prevented a single case of cervical cancer (let alone cervical cancer death), nor that the current overly optimistic surrogate marker-based extrapolations are justified".

"Likewise, the notion that HPV vaccines have an impressive safety profile is only supported by highly flawed design of safety trials and is contrary to accumulating evidence from vaccine safety surveillance databases and case reports which continue to link HPV vaccination to serious adverse outcomes (including death and permanent disabilities)".

"Further reduction of cervical cancers might be best achieved by optimizing cervical screening (which carries no such risks) and targeting other factors of the disease rather than by the reliance on vaccines with questionable efficacy and safety profiles."

***Is the Debate Over?*** — No, the debate on HPV vaccines will continue even though the evidence to effectiveness and safety is yet to be proven clearly. In 2008, Merck spent $93 million to market Gardasil as a vaccine that prevented cervical cancer, a conclusion their clinical trials never reached. However, it is safe to advise that if vaccinated, females should continue to get regular Pap test screening every few years. This is because the HPV vaccines do not protect against all types of cancer causing HPV infections. Pap tests remain the only way to check for abnormal cells.

Exposure to HPV can also occur before any vaccination begins. It is not uncommon for HPV vaccinated women to have an abnormal Pap test. There are many different types of HPV that can contribute and not all may be covered by a vaccine. There is no guarantee that either Gardasil or Cervarix vaccines will prevent cervical cancer.

Again, vaccines do not treat HPV after diagnosis and can be very expensive (Gardasil is administered in three separate doses, each dose retails for $120).

As this book sets out to demonstrate Silver Sol technology instead, utilizes a quantum holistic approach (safer) and in many ways more beneficial. Vaccines for HPV have not yet proven their effectiveness nor have they been proven completely safe at this time. Maybe silver sol technology, used in a complimentary integrated manner with vaccines and condoms, could help turn the tide of HPV infection? A quantum and holistic approach utilizing silver sol gel (along with sound sexual practices) can be a viable alternative to just vaccines for prevention, which remains highly controversial.

# Chapter 4:
# HISTORY OF SILVER IN MEDICINE

***History of Silver*** — So if vaccines are controversial, what if we could introduce a noninvasive and nontoxic complimentary protocol to HPV prevention and treatment? A quantum and holistic approach using something called "silver-sol technology" without side effects? We can. It all begins with an element known as silver.

First let's explore the history of a non-toxic heavy metal called silver. This, for thousands of years, has a medicinal and preservative use around the globe. Throughout man's history, silver was used to discourage pathogens long before the discovery of antibiotics. Much of the following can be found in multiple sources including www.silverhealthinstitute.com.

The ancient Greek civilization learned to use the metal silver in their drinking vessels to purify water sources. Hippocrates, the famous Greek physician and father of modern medicine wrote that "silver could prevent disease and had special healing properties".

The ancient Roman culture also crafted silver utensils out of silver metals to protect themselves from food born bacteria.

The ancient Phoenicians stored liquids in silver lined vessels to deter spoilage.

Have you ever heard of the saying for affluence, "born with a silver spoon in his mouth"? During the plaques of Europe, wealthy families gave their children silver spoons to suck on to protect them from disease.

In the 17th century, American pioneers crossing the vast western expanse, found out that dropping silver coins into their milk containers prevented bacterial growth like tuberculosis. They also used silver in their water containers to prevent dysentery. This was extremely beneficial since they had no refrigeration and municipal filtration.

In the early 19th century dairy farmers often used silver milk pails to retard bacterial growth and contamination.

Also in the 19th century surgeons used silver sutures to close surgical wounds; prevent infection, and to speed up the healing process.

Silver leaf was applied to soldier's wounds during World War I. Silver solutions were used as a topical antiseptic, oral, and even injected intravenously, during World War II.

Prior to the introduction of chemical based antibiotics, colloidal silver was widely used in Hospitals. By 1940 there were 48 identified compounds (FDA approved) of silver used to treat every infectious disease known to man. It was available in oral, injectable, and topical form known as Albargin and Silvol (16).

Currently, Ayurveda medicine uses silver as a tonic or elixir for those suffering from age or debilitating disease consuming nearly 275,000 kg (650,000 lbs.) of edible metallic silver foil every year. They wrap some food and candy (to prevent spoilage) in thin foil and literally consume the whole thing!

The Swiss army uses silver to treat their water today.

Some international airlines use silver as a disinfectant for potable water.

Humidifiers use something called "silver clean technology" embedded in tank of those humidifiers, to discourage mildew and mold.

Silver-plated Foley catheters are used in today's hospitals to prevent urinary tract infection. The metal's bactericidal properties make it ideal for stents and prosthetic implants as well.

The U.S. military weaves silver into undergarments to reduce odor and prevent infection in the field.

NASA uses silver for purification of air and water on board Space Shuttles and Space Stations (17).

Silver nitrate is still used in some hospitals today in a few states for newborn infants, in the eyes to deter syphilis/gonorrhea.

Silver is also used in electrical ionization to help sanitize the water in swimming pools without harsh effects of chlorine. This also explains the historical practice of throwing silver coins into public fountains.

The use of Silver even went to a subcommittee of the U.S. Congress (18).

Even the New York City board of physicians gave its stamp of approval for silver's use as a homeopathic medicine.

Silver itself is one of the best conductors of energy in the entire periodic table of elements.

Reputable labs at the University of Georgia, Kansas State University, Penn State, Arizona State, University of Arizona, University of California at Davis, and Brigham Young University have all completed research supporting silver's use in fighting pathogen infection (19).

Lastly, according to the Merck Manual of Diagnosis and Therapy, silver is not considered to be a heavy metal or to accumulate. It is the only metal not considered to be a heavy metal because it does not produce heavy metal poisoning (20).

***Argyria*** — However, even though silver is not considered a heavy metal. A condition known as "Argyria" has been widely publicized. The only known and recorded adverse health effect ever recorded from use of silver is "Argyria or Argyrosis".

This can only result from using impure silver (less than 99.9% pure elemental) to begin with. It has only been noted to come from questionable manufacturers in the past or using "in home" colloidal silver making devices. Argyria can result in patches of blue or blue-grayish skin, conjunctiva discolor, and even generalized all over the body dis-colorization. It is believed to be irreversible, but not physically harmful.

Since the 1990's "colloidal silver" has been advised against by Medical authorities. However, there has never been a reported case of Argyria from modern "colloidals". There have been instances from using homemade silver devices (21).

### *The Silver Atom (2-8-18-18-1):*

The silver atom has an atomic structure that consists of five orbitals. There are 2, 8, 18, 18 and 1 electrons orbiting in these orbitals. This atomic structure illustrates that silver can accept electrons and conduct energy easily.

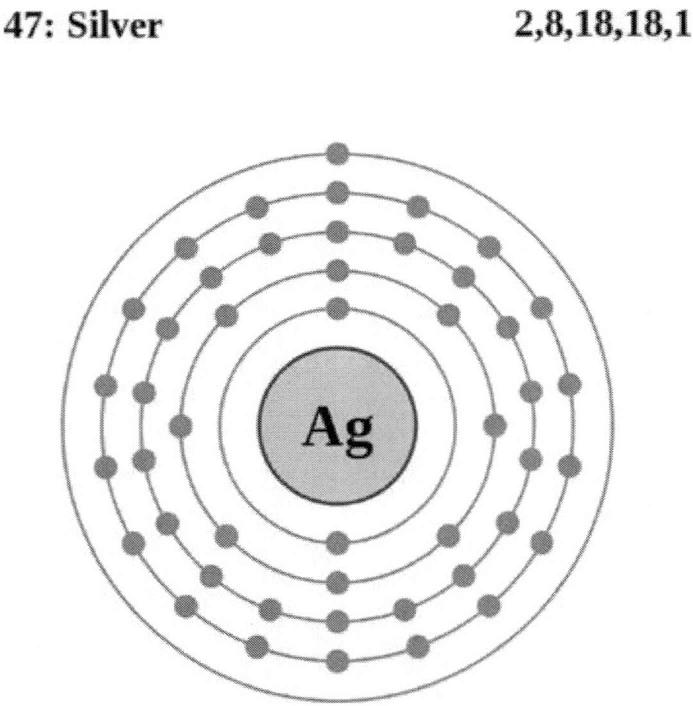

Chapter 5:
# THIS IS NOT YOUR GRANDMOTHER'S SILVER – SILVER SOL TECHNOLOGY

***Colloidal Silver*** — A comparative distinction needs to be addressed describing "colloidal silver" versus a newer "silver sol" technology.

In 1924 the first patent for silver was issued for an older technology called "colloidal silver". A colloid is a particle between 1 and 1000 nanometers in diameter. A nanometer is a unit of length noted as 1 billionth of a meter. It is denoted by the symbol 'nm'.

Colloidal refers to a fine dispersion of silver metal particles into water by using electricity (9 volts of DC). Colloidal silvers have been around for over 100 years. Most commercial silvers still using 1924 technology today have dispersions in the range of 300 to 300,000 part per million. Parts per million (ppm) is a common term for describing the amount of dissolved particles of silver within water. This is done by measuring the mass of dissolved silver in comparison to the mass of the water. Using pure elemental silver (99.99%) to begin with, can help ensure anti-bacterial effectiveness and safety.

Einstein mentioned the term "colloidal" (Brownian Motion Paper) in 1905. He found that "a colloid acts like an atom". This implied the structure and function of even water itself. So the topic of colloidal is important in understanding silver solutions. In Einstein's day, there were three Nobel's given out for colloidal research, two in one year. However, colloidal in Einstein's day, is not the same as the new silver technology of today.

This old colloidal technology often produces brown or yellow looking liquids or gels. It uses far more silver than current technology and is shown to be less effective than the current as well.

Old colloidal silvers tend to "fall out" of suspension and can stick or clump together over time. Again, poor colloids are the chief contributor to the condition known as Argyria. Colloidal silvers tend to have a strong metallic flavor when tasted. They tend to be anti-pathogenic. They do this by "inhibiting" pathogens. Common colloidal (ionic) silver solutions have particles that = -1 electron. This gives the suspended silver particle the ability to bind itself with and eliminate one electron of a targeted pathogen. This helps explain its therapeutic action on inhibition of a pathogen. In simplicity, it takes one colloidal silver particle to take out one pathogen.

***Silver Sol*** — The newer technology (which has a working patent in 2006) is known as "silver sol or aqua sol" silver. Some manufacturers will refer to this new technology with many marketing names such as ionic, hydrosol, aqua sol, or even nano-silver. It will be referred to henceforth, as "Silver sol". This is truly, not your Grandmothers silver.

It has been proven to have no known side effects (19). It will easily pass out of the body unchanged, even in the presence of Hydrochloric acid (HCL), which can bind with any type of silver products to make silver chloride.

The newer silver sol technology is very different from the old colloidal form. It is made with something called "supercharging" (see below). This is a quantum leap in silver technology. Silver sol technology is composed of 0.001 percent pure metallic silver and 99.999 percent water. Again, having pure silver ensures no impurities are transferred or accumulated in the process to those using it. This supercharged liquid silver sol becomes a simple, but powerful, anti-pathogenic solution. Let's break this down further.

"Sol" is also a chemical designation of any pure mineral, permanently suspended in water. The mineral's charge is transferred to the entire body of water. This process of creating a "sol" gives the water a differing structure. The Silver Sol is clear and colorless compared to a colloidal. It is known to actually kill bacteria versus inhibition. It has been shown to help protect Humans against bacteria, viruses, mold, food poisoning, and is a valuable aid in wound healing including burns (22). This technology is available as both a liquid and a gel. The silver sol gel, based on constituents, may have a differing pH than silver sol liquid.

***Supercharging*** — Silver sol uses 10,000 volts of alternating current (AC) rather than 9 volts of direct current (DC). It is AC current that has been found to supercharge the silver. This is an important distinction from the old technology of DC current. This results in a solution that has different atomic structure than a colloid.

Because of this supercharging, Silver (aqua) sol technology has particles which = -2 electrons. This results in an element known as Ag404. This element particle has the ability to bind itself with, and destroy electrons of targeted pathogens, multiple times. The two missing electrons (in the outer shell) give silver catalytic capability. Think of it as one electron is destroying a pathogen (virus), while the other electron is recharging. So you get a "destroy and recharge" happening instantaneously. The result is this silver sol can destroy thousands of times more pathogens, than a simple one electron colloid can do. You get a lot more effect on pathogens, with less part per million (ppm) of supercharged silver in a solution. The supercharging gives specific electron configuration which is better understood by physics than biochemistry. Non acidic, non-ionic, and uses structured water.

***Comparison of Silvers*** — Silver sols have been shown by researchers at Brigham Young University (19) to be highly bioavailable compared to the old colloidal technology. Many old colloids (300-300,000 ppm) on the market were tested by BYU against the new silver sols (in dispersions of only 10-15 ppm). The old colloid technology showed a 15% to 65% bioavailability, depending on manufacturing. The new technology silver solution (sol) exceeded 99% bio-availability. Keep in mind it is due to the -2 electron supercharging, more parts per million (ppm) is not as relevant, such as colloids claim to be. With the new technology more ppm does not equate to a "stronger" silver solution. Bioavailability is way more relevant (see mechanisms of action), which means we can get more action even with less ppm.

This new technology, subject's pure elemental silver to tremendous amounts of energy (AC or supercharging). This tremendous amount of energy will actually "dissolve" silver into water, making the particles extremely small. By this process, the particles are small enough that they are able to retain an electric charge while being permanently suspended in water. The water molecules themselves become more structured ensuring less imperfections. This ensures no fall out or "clumping" like old colloidal silver technology.

The silver sol particles are so small that they are tiny enough to enter a single red blood cell (19). In fact, being 0.05 nm in size, you could fit 2,000 of these silver particles inside a single red blood cell (23).

Silver sol has even demonstrated an ability to make prescription antibiotics more effective. It helps to create synergy in prescription antibiotics and improve the prescription potential in destroying pathogens with uptake (24). Silver sol can help take the burden off the immune system by assisting pathogen destruction with antibiotics. This is the essence of integrative medicine.

It has even been demonstrated to have the ability to destroy malarial parasites in the erythrocytic phase. In research done in Ghana, Africa silver sol safely and completely removed the malaria parasite from the blood in 100% of 56 human subjects infected with malaria in an average of five days (25). It is a known cure for malaria (25, 26).

Silver sol is small enough and safe enough to consume internally or apply topically every day. If Einstein were alive, he would definitely have an expanded his view of colloidal with the new silver sol technology.

***Colloidal vs. Silver Sol*** — An ion is an atom or molecule with an unequal number of protons and electrons. Ions can have a positive or negative charge to them. In a comparative bacteriology analysis using particulate silver (colloid) versus silver sol (ionic), an experiment proved that silver in ionic form, is where the antibacterial property of silver truly resides (27).

Silver sol will leave the body unchanged (un-metabolized) and is virtually nontoxic. Again, colloidal silvers can be toxic, as evidenced from homemade machines producing a condition of Argyria. Research has shown 98 percent of all silver sol ingested, leaves the body within twenty four hours (19). It has been considered safe enough for age 6 months old, to all the way to end of life care.

Additional properties of silver sol are being discovered all the time. Including anti-inflammatory properties, which works by eliminating pathogens, in turn decreases inflammation. This allows the body to focus on healing instead of fighting chronic inflammation. It has immune enhancement properties by taking the stress off the immune system, because of dealing with pathogen infection. It is cost effective (versus cost of allopathic prescriptions). A 4 oz. tube of silver sol gel (24ppm) is around $30.00 ($ U.S.).

***Images of Silver*** — The following images are pictures of silver binding with purified water molecules at a moment in time. The first image shows silver (Ag) molecules binding with water in a beaker. Notice the columns of silver sol coming off the coil of pure silver at the base of the beaker. As AC current is passed thru the silver coil, silver ions bind with hydrogen bonds to form silver sol. This image frozen in time shows literally the molecules of silver sol forming creating molecules of Ag406, Ag404, Ag202, and Ag204.

The second image has a laser shown thru it, demonstrating what is known as the "tindle" effect.

*(Pictures reprinted with permission from Dr. Gordon Pederson)*

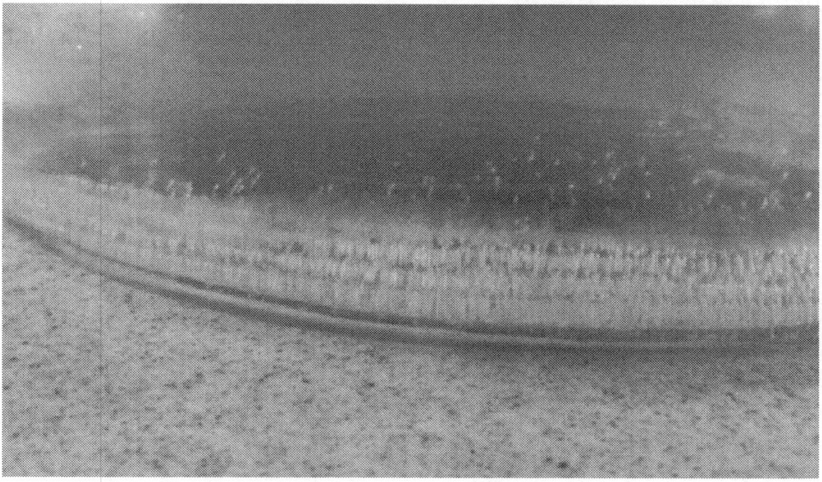

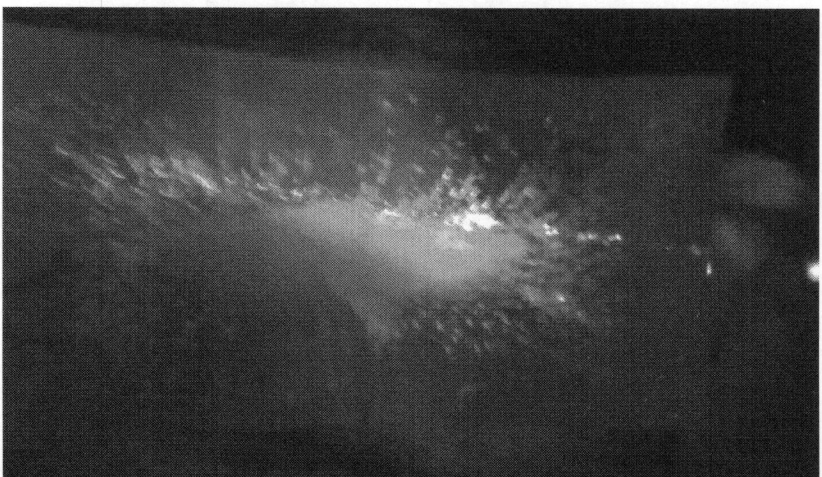

***Silver Sol Function*** — Once silver sol (liquid) is made, it can be added to a carbomer to make a gel form.

The silver sol gel form (24ppm), functions similar to an antibiotic (more or less equal to pharmaceutical drugs), but is unique because bacteria do not mutate or become resistant to this form of silver (28). In China, India, and some other countries silver sol derivatives are often used in traditional medicine as an antibacterial and antiviral.

There are many uses of silver sol gel worth mentioning, other than HPV application. It can be applied to sunburn, used for skin health, a hand sanitizer, wound care, and as a personal lubricant.

In the case of other antiviral activity, silver sol technology has been used against viruses like HIV-1 (29 -32), Hepatitis B virus (33), Monkey Pox virus (34), Tacaribe virus (35), Influenza virus (36), Herpes Simplex virus (37) and Respiratory Syncytial virus (38).

In one study, using something called a MTT method, it showed that silver sol preparations of concentrations less than 100ug/ml, inhibited replication of the HSV-2 virus. This helped demonstrate silver sol as a promising use against sexually transmitted diseases (39). Again, this is not your Grandmothers Silver (colloidal).

Only one contraindication exists with use of any silver sol is saline. The salts in a solution can inactivate the silver sol. The chloride ion binds with silver particles. So if taking silver sol internally, do so on an empty stomach to keep away from salty foods or medication. Same with the silver sol gel form, keeping salt away from the gel, such as in the case of a saline douche.

In conclusion, the distinction between the old and new technology, the super charged silver sol is showing more benefits, safety, all at much lower concentrations (5-40 ppm) than colloids. Silver sol derives its power from three primary mechanisms of action.

Chapter 6:
# THE MECHANISMS OF ACTION OF SILVER SOL TECHNOLOGY

Silver (Ag406, Ag404, Ag202, and Ag204) whether in liquid or gel form, can help destroy bacteria, viruses, some parasites and fungi, through a combination of mechanisms.

***Chemical Structure/Contact*** — As noted above (supercharging) is = -2 electrons. Due to this chemical structure, it has this ability to destroy multiple pathogens with less ppm of silver. To be extremely effective it must have contact time with a pathogen. Contact time requires about 5-12 minutes with pathogens, which will help ensure destruction. Some pathogens require more minutes than others based on studies. So in general we will say 10-12 minutes to help ensure a broad spectrum appeal. Silver sol binds to the surface of a pathogen covalently by stealing an electron from the membrane of that pathogen. This results in lysis of the pathogen membrane. This is a redox reaction taking place, which is chemical reaction.

The redox reaction is a recurring, cyclical silver reaction that consists of two actions. The first is the stealing of an electron from a pathogen. The second consists of firing a high-energy electron back into the pathogen. This reaction takes place in approximately one ten thousandth of a second. The results are devastating to the cellular membrane of a disease-causing pathogen. It is because the silver sol steals an electron, rupturing the pathogen, and immediately can fire an electron back into it. As long as the silver steals electrons, it will always fire an equal amount back. So, when an electron is stolen from a pathogen, the pathogen is oxidized and the silver is reduced resulting in a ruptured bacterial membrane of the pathogen and energized silver.

This give and take reaction is that there are only as many electrons fired at the bonded pathogen as there are stolen electrons. This mechanism is what differentiates what happens in colloidal or even old ionic silvers (colloidal and older forms of silver are limited to the removal of a single pathogenic electron, non-supercharged). Again, this is why colloidal and older ionic versions of silver require a concentration consisting of hundreds of thousands of ppm to kill as many pathogens as silver sols do with far less ppm.

Silver sols chemical structure continues to kill as long as it removes an electron. It can recharge and fire back without consuming or neutralizing the oxygenated silver. This results in unique silver that has continuous killing capacity (a catalytic reaction).

This redox reaction can also help mediate pain because it removes an electron from the surface protein of pain receptors. This redox reaction minimizes inflammation and transmission of the pain response within the pain receptors. Supercharged silver exchanges electrons between molecules and atoms resulting in numerous modes of action. Chemical structure and contact time is just the beginning.

Tetrahedral shapes (i.e. Ag 202, 204 etc.) form and work because of the electromagnetic energy produced by the transfer of silver ions within the molecule. So in using silver sols with people one must be fundamentally creative (new meaning of an old context). It may involve "how you can get it in direct contact with pathogens". For example, in cases of respiratory disorders, you may want to add liquid silver sol to a nebulizer for inhalation, to ensure contact time with pathogens in the lungs.

***Resonance or Frequency (Magnetic Disruption)*** — remember Royal Raymond Rife and his Rife microscope?

Rife identified spectroscopic signatures to microbes and viruses. He used a slit spectroscope attached to his microscope. Then he slowly rotated a quartz prism focusing light of a single wave-length onto the viruses he was looking at.

It is a known fact that every molecule oscillates at its own distinct frequency. He selected a wave-length that resonated with the signature frequency of a virus. We know atoms come together to form a molecule and are held together in a configuration with a covalent energy bond. This bond emits and absorbs its own specific electromagnetic frequency. No two molecules have the same signature or frequency. By using this wavelength resonance Rife helped make the invisible (virus), visible.

He could now observe a live virus actively invading tissue cultures. Most small organisms like viruses are only visible with ultraviolet light which is outside the human eye spectrum. Rife perfected a technique called heterodyning. He did this by illuminating the virus with two different wavelengths of the same ultraviolet light frequency. These resonated with the signature of the virus. The two wavelengths produced interference when they merged like waves of an ocean. This interference produced a third visible wave in the electromagnetic spectrum. It made the invisible virus, visible. This cannot even be done with today's electron microscopes.

Rife was an important pioneer in resonance or frequency of a virus. He went on to document this discovery. He even identified a certain virus he was looking at as a cancer virus. He named it Cryptocides Primordiales. He went on to describe that it had a pleomorphic nature which has been validated by dark field techniques of today and also with the Naessen's microscope. So the idea of resonance and frequency comes into play here.

Rife used the same principles he discovered to kill viruses, by resonance. By increasing the intensity of a frequency that resonated with the virus, he increased the frequency oscillation until the virus exploded. The interesting thing to note is it did no damage to healthy surrounding tissues. Quantum physics tells us that everything, down to its smallest component is simply energy vibrating at a specific frequency. Rife may have been using Quantum medicine?

Silver sol can also cause viral replication interference with this same concept of resonance and frequency. Silver sol can bond with a virus through magnetic and electrical resonance. The resonant frequency of the silver sol then results in the disruption of the virus.

The silver in suspension (sol) is multi-phasic. It is known as a di-electro-magnetic semi-conductor. So it will produce a resonant frequency. It is similar to a tiny nano-electrocution (23). This nano-electrocution interferes with a virus's ability to attach to host cells.

The tetrahedral silver sol particles are missing two electrons and have been identified as silver II oxide (40), because the Ag4O4 consists of a crystalline structured molecule that has two different charges (1+ and 3+), it is by definition a multi-phasic, divalent semi-conductor of electro-magnetic energy.

This unique molecule produces a magnetic field and an electrical wavelength that together are capable of destroying pathogens while it is being transported ubiquitously throughout circulation.

The Merck Manual (20) identifies Silver II Oxide as consisting of four atoms of oxygen and four atoms of silver bonded in a crystalline structure where two of the silver atoms have a 1+ (monovalent charge, missing one electron) and the other two atoms of silver have a 3+ (trivalent charge, missing three electrons).

There is a high energy particle (electron) that continuously moves at quantum speed between the monovalent and trivalent silver atoms, and when measured by instrumentation gives off an overall charge of 2+. Ag4O4 is identified as a Silver II Oxide missing two electrons in its outer valence, and historically this is the label placed upon Ag4O4, but it is significant to the mechanism of actions to recognize that silver is actually a molecule with two different charges.

The 1+ and 3+ charges exist on the same molecule and perform as a di-electro-magnet with an electric wavelength and a magnetic field that together destroy disease-causing pathogens.

In practice, a testimonial letter from a medical doctor reported the effective use of silver sol in more than 50 cases involving patients with viral pneumonia. The testimony also includes many other pathogens such as HIV and Herpes Zoster (41).

### ***Cellular Frequency*** —

"The cell is a machine driven by energy. It can thus be approached by studying matter, or by studying energy. In every culture and in every medical tradition before ours, healing was accomplished by moving energy."

— Albert Szent-Gyorgyi (Nobel Laureate in Medicine)

Cells have the unique ability to store countless numbers of frequencies in their cytoplasm. Hydrogen and Oxygen hold electromagnetic charges within the cell. It is processed as cellular memory within the DNA of each cell. This is all part of the homeostasis of the cell.

Prolonged and undealt with stress (physical, emotional, mental) increases the cells vulnerability to disruptive frequency. Even a cell phone (EMF) or microwaves can enter a cells cytoplasm and alter frequency. Every negative emotion, pathogen, or disease state, has its own frequency and can alter cellular function.

A virus pathogen (HPV) can introduce an associated harmonic frequency of its own which becomes disharmonic to the once healthy cell.

Royal Raymond Rife (1888-1971) was ultimately dismissed as a "quack" by the AMA and FDA but again, he did help pioneer energy medicine. He firmly believed that different species of life have their own electromagnetic signatures. In 1934 he opened a clinic that successfully cured 16 of 16 cancer cases within 3 months. He attributed the cause of these cases to disharmonious viral frequency. He found that the cancer virus could be destroyed by the use of electromagnetic frequency (42). Biophysics today uses magnetism, wavelengths (MRI's), and energy.

Scientifically we know the majority of most pathogens resonate at a frequency of about 890-910 terahertz. These frequencies are also similar to germicidal ultraviolet light bulbs used in hospitals. This is used to denature germs for anti-septic reasons. I used to work in surgery in my early career at a hospital and noticed these ultraviolet lights everywhere. Similarly, silver sol resonates at that those same frequencies as pathogens. In the case of a virus, silver sol then can actually suppress and contain viral infection by interfering with the duplication and replication with frequency. Simply, the frequencies attract, and so doing, cancel each other out. The virus becomes inactivated.

Silver sol frequency works against both reverse transcriptase and DNA polymerase virus. It is important to note again, that contact time increases the potency of stopping replication. The more mechanisms of action you can use with silver sol, the better the outcome. The closer you can get "magnets" together, the better the attraction! You want to get silver sol gel in direct areas with where the virus is located. As in the case of HPV, use of a tampon coated with silver sol gel. Insert it into the vagina in direct proximity of HPV and the cervix for women. This is usually inserted for about 30 minutes to ensure contact time and resonance. It can be used up to four times a day, four hours apart. It is done in the case studies protocol for seven days straight.

Now, a virus is constructed of something called a capsid. This capsid (a microscopic cellular container) is a protein shell and or lipid membrane, enclosing the genetic material segments of the virus. Inside the capsid are incomplete segments of DNA and RNA. The virus (referred to previously as a tangled hierarchy) can bind to a healthy cellular surface. Through fusion it injects these incomplete segments of DNA or RNA. The segments themselves however, carry a slight magnetic charge. Hence, contact time of silver sol (magnetic disruption) increases the effectiveness of silver as an anti-viral.

The capsid has an external mechanism to assemble a stable, protective protein shell to protect the insides of the virus from lethal chemical and physical agents. These agents include forms like natural radiation, extremes of pH or temperature, proteolytic and nucleolytic enzymes (43).

Once the virus attaches to a host cell, it injects its segments causing damage to the healthy cell. This results in abnormal reproduction of once normal cells or disease. This also causes once healthy cells to divide abnormally. Just one virus can produce up to 10,000 more copies of the virus (using the once healthy cell) that bud off or rupture. This scatters the virus to other cells throughout the whole area or body (44).

Silver sol works with resonance (magnet) to charged DNA particles from the virus, so that the silver will bind to those segments. This prevents the segments from stretching out and then the virus cannot replicate. It basically makes the virus inactive. The DNA segments are now so tightly bound to the silver sol particle ion that the genetic material can no longer go through the replication process.

As you can see silver sol has many diverse levels of activity, and has received numerous approved patents from the United States Patent office. They include anti-viral (19), anti-microbial (19), anti-fungal (19), and bubonic plague (45) while sparing the good probiotic bacteria (46). This is very unique technology that it spares our good bacteria. It is because our probiotic bacteria have a much thicker capsid or membrane and a more balanced charge. This results in a different frequency than pathogens. This helps protect not only the good bacteria but also our healthy cells exhibit the same thing. Normal healthy cells are not resonating to the supercharged silver's magnetic attraction. Therefore, the silver sol does not bind with healthy cellular DNA. It will only bind with the viral frequency that the silver sol is similar in. This makes silver sol selective only to certain frequencies of pathogens, which resonate at that same frequency (890-910 terahertz). Beneficial bacteria (probiotics) resonate at a much different frequency (47) and therefore are not magnetically resonant to silver sol. Probiotics bacteria also have a double layer (fat) membrane, were pathogens (water based) usually do not. The "aha" moment here is: know any prescription antibiotic that can do that? To emphasize, although mentioned previously, silver sol has even been published as a cure for malaria (25).

***Cellular Communication*** — Another mechanism of action is cellular communication. Most cells communicate with each other by an outside sugary coating. This type of coating lets a cell know who is friend or who is a foe. Pathogens use this process as well to detect white blood cells which has an unfriendly coating.

Silver sol has "friendly" sugar coating. This helps make it attractive to pathogens or even an abnormal cell, after all cells love sugar. Silver sol then interferes with replication of that pathogen only (after frequency and resonance). In theory, it makes it very hard for pathogens to become "resistant" to something that is so yummy.

*An illustration of a viral replication process without silver sol:*

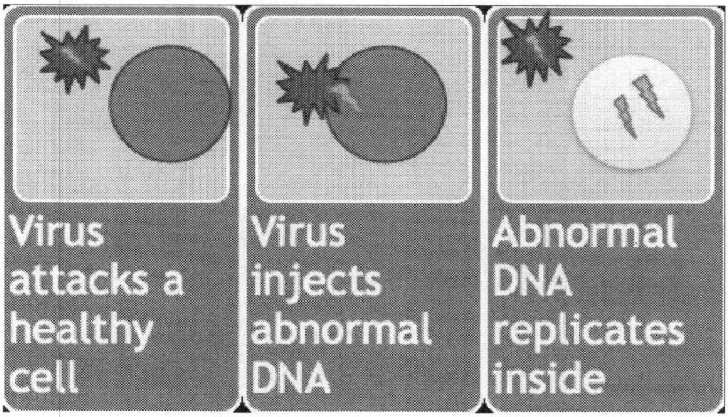


The above viral process repeats again and again, resulting in infection.

*An illustration of deterring viral replication with Silver Sol:*

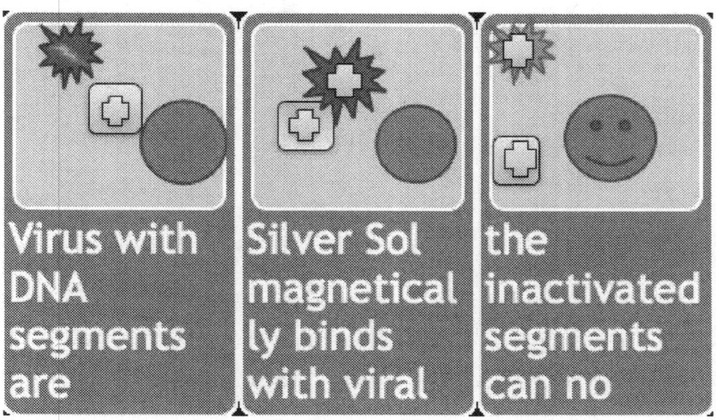

These are just a few of the main mechanisms of action but give a very clear picture of how this technology can be used in the interfering of a HPV infection.

This is why so many uses of silver have been approved and patents issued. Silver sol is even EPA certified for odors/foods (48).

Silver is also considered a regenerative product. It does this by helping the body to heal quicker. By lessening the immune burden duties of having to first destroy pathogens, which get in the way of healing of any tissue.

# Chapter 7:
# ADVANCEMENT OF SILVER SOL TECHNOLOGY TODAY

Since silver sol is relatively new, advancements keep happening even as of this writing. It is worth addressing and mentioning that this type of quantum medicine is ever improving.

***Structured Water*** — Another advent to the silver sol technology is something called "structured water". Structured water is defined as a "hexagonal water" structure or cluster, like what is found in snow water. It has been postulated that structured water may help with cellular communication. Although many incompatibilities exist with modern science, we do know that in the homeopathic principles from Samuel Hahnemann (father of homeopathy), that water is the universal carrier of frequency (resonance). The more pure a water source is (point of origin), the better a carrier for the homeopathic remedy. In this case, silver sol.

So by studying the structure of water we can find advances in technology of silver sol (which is 99.999% water).

Professor Rustum Roy, who held five professorships at various universities, showed that temperature and pressure are not the only things that effect water structure. He lectured for years that electric fields, magnetic fields, and strain fields, can change waters structure too. He championed the science term "epitaxy". This is where an imprint from one structure, will transfer onto another without transferring any matter itself, especially from a solid to a liquid. An example of this is semiconductors (49).

Silver sol is an example of changing the waters structure just by suspending supercharged silver nanoparticles. The silver suspended minerals have strong electrostatic fields around it. This can be epitaxial itself. Water is considered the universal carrier of everything in it. It can carry sound, acoustics, and vibrations. Why couldn't it carry in its structure subtle energies or even intent?

For example consider homeopathy. Modern science tends to dismiss homeopathy as a joke. Yet it is an example of structured water itself. A water preparation of a deluded substance that is even diluted to the point of having nothing left of the original substance. But anyone who has ever used homeopathy and healed themselves of a condition, would argue. This is especially true with homeopathic use in animals, which do not subscribe to placebo effect. But yet the energy of the homeopathic has been shown to return animals to homeostasis. This is vibrational medicine at its best. Even water tumbling out of a faucet is structured differently every time, each second as it falls.

Experimental observations of structured water clusters require spectroscopic tools such as infrared spectroscopy, vibration-rotation-tunneling (VRT) and Far-infrared, just to name a few. But these types of tools do confirm this idea of structured water, even help prove epitaxial influence. The evidence, even if some is anecdotal, about silver sol structured water is indisputable.

Dr. Gordon Pedersen, who originally created silver sol, feels very strongly that structured water (pH balanced and pure) is synergistically important to the effectiveness and continued advancement of silver sol technology. Alkaline silver sol (7.4 pH) for internal use and gels has successfully demonstrated electrical activity, magnetic activity, chemical activity, and an increase in the activation and mobilization of immune cells including stem cell activation (50). This is part of the advancement of silver sols today.

***Image:*** *The following is model representation of Silver Ag404 molecule.*

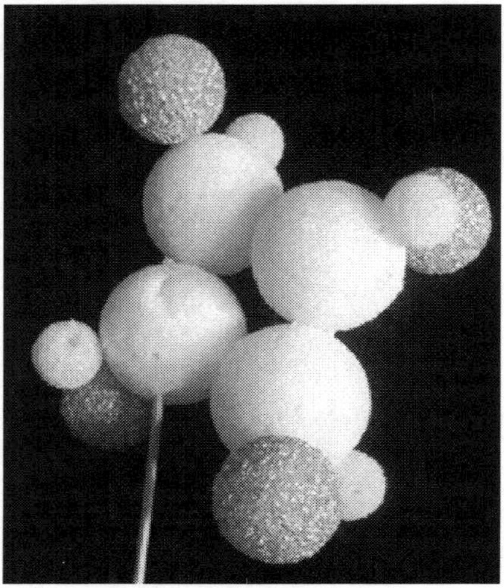

This model helps show the di-electro-magnetic Ag404 molecule. It is a semiconductor that resonates at an antimicrobial frequency or frequencies. There are four water molecules that hold a structure for the four silver atoms to permanently attach.

**Silver sol thru Raman Spectra Analysis.**

Raman Spectra analysis demonstrates a unique graphic representation presenting a pattern different from any other silver, see Graph 1.0 (51). This demonstrates a unique silver pattern.

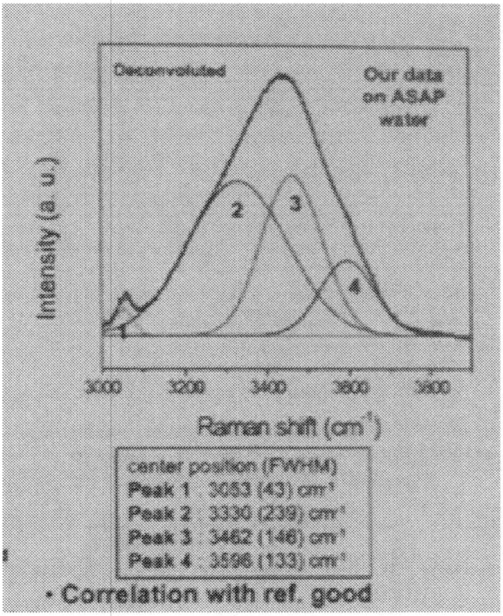


***Graph 1.0** Raman Spectra Analysis*

TEM imaging of Silver Sol (electron microscope):

Electron microscopic images and small area nano-diffraction, demonstrate images that confirm the presence of Ag4O4. Graph 2.0 illustrates broadened and elongated diffraction spots, which indicate a range of distribution of the crystal inter plane distances (51). TEM Image and Small Area Nano-diffraction pattern confirms the presence of Ag404. This electron microscopic image confirms the broad and elongated diffraction spots. This indicates there is distribution of the crystal inter plane distances. This is different than any other silver and helps explain the ability of Silver Sol to expand or contract the nano-silver particle to the needed size or cluster.

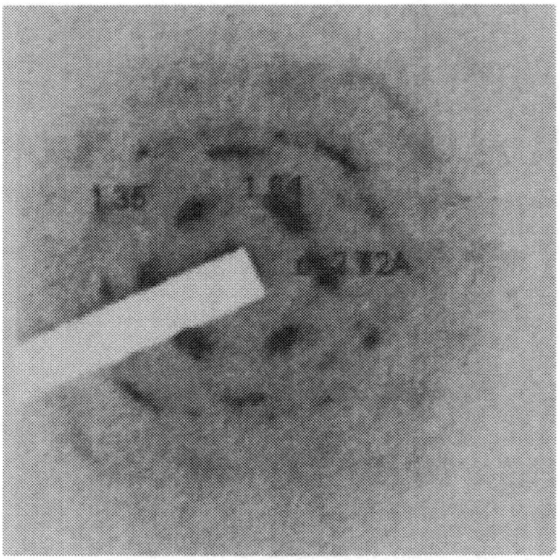

***Graph 2.0*** *TEM image and small area nano diffraction pattern.*

These images continue to pioneer the advancement of silver sol including pH modifications and enhanced structured water.

***Masaru Emoto*** — Going another step further in the understanding of structured water, water crystals themselves play a role in advancement. Dr. Masaru Emoto is a pioneer in water crystal research (52). He has photographed thousands of water crystals and has demonstrated even how water has a unique role in carrying natural vibrations of words. His work is undeniable on the key concept of resonance. He describes in his book "The Miracle of Water" that humans are made up of roughly 70% water in body. His pioneering work helps show that water within us carries vibrations and reflects our language. Positive words will help form beautiful looking photographed water crystals. While negative words form incomplete ugly looking water crystals.

Do Masaru Emoto's pictures lie? They have been confirmed as untouched or edited. Whether we agree with structuring water or not, the above arguments make sense. The simple act of tumbling water out of a faucet has been shown to re-structure water for seconds. In the case of Hahnemann, Pedersen, or Emoto, water as a carrier of resonance is worth mentioning as a quantum approach in advancement of silver sol.

***Silver and Gold*** — Gold nanoparticles are now being considered along with silver sol and structured waters. Gold nanoparticles have already been used by traditional cancer doctors. They use it because gold particles can be absorbed into tiny cellular spaces. They act as an anti-inflammatory, while simultaneously bonding with an anticancer drug. This helps deliver the gold and drug into damaged and inflamed tissues as well (53). The gold will also bond with silver sol particles working to not only reduce pathogens, but become anti-inflammatory. Gold is known to have little or no toxicity, resistance, and even help carry supplements to tissues (54). Advancements in this area are already happening.

# Chapter 8:
# SILVER SOL TECHNOLOGY AND SUPERBUGS

Paul K. Carlton Jr., who served as the Surgeon General of the Air Force from 1999-2002 and currently serves as Director of Integrative Center for Homeland Security at Texas A&M, stated this about silver sol: "In short, we currently do not have anything with such a wide spectrum of efficacy…in our inventory."

Even against super bugs (i.e. overuse of antibiotics) silver sol offers a safe and effective means of fighting pathogens, like viruses, where other drugs may fail. It shows promise in protecting us from epidemic outbreaks, contagions, and bio-terrorist attacks.

May 17th 2014 the CDC reported the first evidence of MERS (Middle East Respiratory Syndrome) coronavirus in the U.S. It already has infected 530 people worldwide and killed 145. The CDC reports that it spread from one person to another inside the U.S. – possibly from a handshake. This is one example of a superbug, most likely a crossover from animals. Superbugs and mutated viruses crossing over from animals are on the increase and will continue. There currently are no drugs or vaccines for MERS. But consider silver sol as a trial, it is known to help curb viral replication.

One big superbug most of us know is MRSA. On any given day there are 30,000 new cases of Methicillin Resistant Staphylococcus Aureus (MRSA). More than 95% of all staphylococcus aureus bacterium are resistant to penicillin. 60% of staph bacteria are also resistant to the replacement antibiotic called methicillin. This has resulted in a strain of superbug known as MRSA. This is a very virulent organism with high survival. Time magazine in July 2014 had a small article on how scientists cultured airplane tables and discovered they had E. coli and MRSA on them. They proved the MRSA could survive in the porous table surface for up to eight days. How many people sit at those tables every day?

Silver sol can be a go-to for superbugs. It can be so effective in pathogen destruction that BYU demonstrated that just 2.5-5.0ppm of silver sol has been shown to be effective in inhibiting or killing MRSA (22). Silver has shown up in multiple references for wound care as well, which MRSA is highly watched out for, as it is so difficult to allopathically treat (55). According to JAMA (Oct. 2007) MRSA accounted for 94,360 serious infections, 18,650 hospital-stay related deaths (56).

Kenneth Friedman Ph.D. from M.I.T. stated this "Based on my research, I have found this new silver solution to be safe and effective weapon against harmful yeasts, viruses, and bacteria. Its low concentration, high effectiveness, and lack of side effects make it an ideal supplement for the prevention and care of conditions associated with these pathogens."

According to the Surgeons Scrub Test protocol, silver aqua sol gel was found to kill 99.999 % of all pathogens for a total of four hours (57). It has been estimated most anti-microbial soaps only last 20 minutes.

Additional study and research on silver aqua sol technology needs to be widened. We know that with the advent of "superbugs" from overuse of antibiotics (i.e. MRSA) and cross over pathogens from animals (i.e. Avian Bird Flu H5N1, Swine flu), that current allopathic remedies are lacking. In the U.S. alone, roughly 2 million people every year get infections that can't be treated with antibiotics and 23,000 of them die as a result (56).

According to the World Health Organization in 2014 in some countries, 50% of people infected with K. pneumonia or E. coli bacteria won't respond to even the most powerful antibiotics. This was revealed as a worldwide serious threat to public health (58). Bacteria and viruses continue to evolve resistance. Super bugs like HDM-1, KPC, and MERS-CoV have all been in the news recently and pose serious threats to all, especially healthcare workers. The wide spread use of anti-microbial soaps and sanitizers, over- prescribed antibiotics, rampant use of antibiotics in livestock, are all creating a need for a more quantum holistic approach to pathogens. Silver aqua sol can help integrate the way.

Silver sol gel functions as an antibiotic more or less equal to pharmaceutical drugs. Because it is unique, bacteria do not mutate or become resistant to this form of Silver (24). Is that not how we should treat superbugs?

Silver sol has even been demonstrated to be a powerful adjunct in surgery to help decrease possible hospital acquired infections (superbugs) during healing of bone surgeries (59, 60).

As with women health issues, many gynecological problems often accompany MD visits, such as a yeast infection with accompanying burning and itching. Powerful anti-fungals are then given. We don't need super-yeast too. This often occurs after a course of antibiotics which diminish good bacteria in the vaginal body and allow fungus to proliferate. Yeast over proliferate in the vagina which is a warm moist area. A study at University Of California at Davis found silver aqua sol to be effective against the yeast S. cerevisiae variant Montrachet (61). Candida albicans was also inhibited.

Regular and preventative use with silver sol gel may help stem the tide of superbugs. Could HPV mutate to more virulent form? Of course, so in the bedroom it can be used as a personal vaginal lubricant. By now you may be thinking this should be in every bedroom everywhere period. Silver has been shown to be beneficial for gynecological infections (62). It helps by interfering with HPV virus in the early phases. As with all viruses, the infection continues to duplicate and becomes much more difficult to control, if left to erupt. As stated earlier, many times women (and men) may be asymptomatic with HPV. The evolution of this virus will continue. We carry the virus and are exposing others/partners to the virus without knowing it, or before the virus is detected by PAP. For men, it can reside mostly in the folds of the uncircumcised penis.

# Chapter 9: CERVICAL CANCER IS N A DISEASE, BUT A SYMPT

***"Why Me"?*** — Cervical cancer, which HPV is a known cause, is truly an expression of dis-ease from an infection, undetected. It is a symptom of a much larger under lying imbalance or even thought of as an end product of the HPV infection. It hopefully is also a wake-up call to change one's lifestyle. Most people, when they are told they have a condition (like cervical cancer), may think "why me"?

Well why not you? Crass as this seems, taking responsibility for our health requires determination, acceptance, and an in-depth knowledge, of how we even become ill. As in HPV, knowing how these types of viruses are transmitted is helpful. Also, being able to comprehend that one's human condition was ripe for infection to begin with, helps relieve some of the shock. After all, most HPV infections are just watched until the PAP notes otherwise. By using an integrated quantum and holistic approach, we are truly able to help restore homeostasis or balance and even deter infection from taking place. By helping one's body to help itself. If we take responsibility for our own health, we truly become empowered.

Through a new understanding of why we get sick, are we truly able to affect the outcome. We will by nature, take action, change our lives for the better, if we are willing to learn from how illness even takes place. That cannot be done effectively if the mindset is simply to "fight" a cancer versus addressing the cause. Cervical cancer is a symptom of the cervix tissue that is the end result of an HPV infection which we may have "earned".

The American Cancer Society states on its website: "Cancer starts when cells in a part of the body start to grow out of control." This is obviously different than normal cell growth and division. Instead of normal cells dying thru a regular process, cancer cells continue to grow and proliferate unchecked by the immune system. They can even grow into our other tissues which normal cells do not. In the case of cervical cancer it can spread throughout the uterus, into the fallopian tubes, ovaries, or surrounding ssues. Cells simply become cancerous because of damage to DNA. n't want cells making bad copies of itself from mutated DNA. The NA is what directs the cell in its actions.

Normal cells have three choices, continue normal cellular division (homeostasis), result in apoptosis (programmed cell death - necessary to stop cancer), or uncontrolled abnormal growth (cancer). You don't want the latter.

Typically in HPV infection, and its early stages of cervical cancer, most women do not experience any noticeable symptoms at all. It is normally detected routinely by a Pap smear. Having a regular Pap smear is critical for cervical health assessment. If outwardly symptoms do appear, pay attention to things like abnormal vaginal bleeding or bleeding after intercourse. Pay attention to unusual vaginal discharge which can be described as watery, thick, and/or contain mucus. Abnormal discharge may be foul smelling as well. Other symptoms to pay attention to (consult your doctor/Pap) are pelvic pain which occurs frequently, pain during urination, and/or pain during sex.

People can inherit cell damaged DNA (again not random mutation), but most DNA damage to begin with is caused by changes to it from the environment (HPV) or stress. In the case of cervical cancer, introducing a foreign pathogen (HPV) to the internal environment of the reproductive tract is obvious. In the book, "The Hidden Story of Cancer", Dr. Peskin describes in detail of why cancer happens. He states that no genetic cause will be found for the vast majority of cancers. He believes that cancer is a primitive defense mechanism for survival from an unhealthy internal environment or biological terrain. A symptom if you will.

***Symptom Treatment*** — Treatments of HPV infection (see last chapter) and cancer symptoms can be expensive, invasive, and ineffective. Options are cryosurgery and even in some cases hysterectomy if warranted. Every year we hear of new cancer drugs and promises. Yet, the percentage of Americans dying from all types of cancers is about the same in 2003 as it was in 1970 back when then President Nixon declared a "War on Cancer". At that time 1 out of every 21 Americans were diagnosed. Today in 2015, one out of every two and half Americans is diagnosed. Yes earlier detection, like in the case of HPV testing and Pap smears, are helping save lives. But just look at the website: http://surveillance.cancer.gov/statistics/types/survival.html which chronologically gives us 5 year survival rates and shows very little improvement.

Current Medical research is supposed to be based on 'evidence based medicine'. This was outlined in the vaccine debate chapter and design flaws were exposed. Other times research has been misrepresented or even data suppressed (63, 64). It is not the purpose here to debate this point but to address that alternative or integrated approaches are not even considered! Mostly, this is because the 'evidence base' cannot be done without funding. Many naturals/alternatives are not evidenced based because there is no way to recoup the funding if proven (unless made synthetically or patented for profit). Therefore medical associations (since naturals can't be prescribed anyway - not evidence based) look the other way. Much of the conclusions from using naturals are historical and anecdotal. Integration of these age old naturals is seriously not anti-allopathic. The "us versus them" mentality should not exist anywhere in medicine. It should be about blending the best of both sciences in to a tangled hierarchy, for the betterment of the world (integration). Soundly, silver sol technology has a deep researched track record in efficacy and safety. It meets both criteria of evidence and natural but does it have to be prescribed to be valid? If Epsom salts can be recommended in an allopathic visit, why not silver sol?

***Monomorphism and Pleomorphism*** — Lets just consider conventional allopathic thinking. Based on the work of Louis Pasteur, the theory of mono-morphism became known. Bacteria, viruses, and other microorganisms, were seen as dangerous and pathogenic. Pasteur considered this the true cause of all disease. This thinking has saved many lives with the advent of certain drugs and continues to do so today. Although eventually on his deathbed, he admitted that this was not the case.

Now, let's consider a different creative view (although not relatively new) which throws a wrench in Pasteur logic. Another pioneer, Bechamp (Pierre Antione), promoted the idea of Pleo-morphism. This is the ability of some pathogens to alter their shape or size in response to their environmental conditions. Even certain fungi will morph into different shapes or stages based on environment (see Candida infections). Bechamp radically proposed that microbes can be seen as necessary and serve a "clean up" function to certain tissues of the body. He advocated looking at the environment of the body instead. His logic was environment determines whether or not a pathogen will be dangerous or beneficial. In other words, microbes change or morph into a good or bad thing depending upon the environment they are in. This is today referred to as Biological Terrain (see next chapter). A paradigm shift from infection comes from a pathogen only.

Conventional medicine still tends to adhere to mono-morphism ideas and tends to treat infections with strong antibiotics, antifungals, and antivirals. In contrast, a pleomorphism approach would address the underlying biological terrain, thus deterring pathogens from making a host a home. This does not favor the notion that a pathogen (HPV) takes hold and progresses into cellular changes like cervical cancer with every infection. It starts to become clearer that cervical cancer may be a symptom of the terrain or environment (pleomorphism) versus the HPV infection only (monomorphism).

In relation to this pleomorphism environment concept, even cells who are DNA damaged from a viral infection like HPV will change their respiration process from aerobic to anaerobic fermentation (65). An exception to this is muscle cells. Dr. Otto Warburg, a brilliant Nobel prize-winning scientist argued this fact. If we hope to destroy any abnormal cells, then targeting the environment makes sense. Change the conditions, you change the outcome. Helping change the biological terrain more favorably within the body can ensure an aerobic condition, thus starving out the fermentation (sugar as fuel) process. Cancer is a symptom of a body's inability to manage its own environment. The trick is to make ones internal environment in-hospitable to cervical cancer or HPV infection (pathogen). This can be done by maintaining a balance to the internal environment (biological terrain) to begin with.

## Chapter 10:
# WHAT IS BIOLOGICAL TERRAIN?

***The Terrain Analogy*** — Biological terrain is another way of saying "the human body's internal environment": similar to soil for plants. The better the condition the plant soil is, the less weeds, disease, insects, and mal absorption of nutrients, the plants will have. The plants are only as healthy as the soil they live in. Humans are very similar in this concept. If our soil (internal environment) is poor, then it is ripe for invaders (pathogens) to live in.

In the terrain analogy, again if weeds appear in soil, it is often a sign that the soil itself is poor. So like poor soil, if pathogens appear in humans, it too is a sign that our soil (terrain) is poor. Like Mother Nature, weeds are a way to break down soil components, to help the soil become more biologically healthy. Weeds are nature's garbage collectors and recyclers. In humans, we have multiple systems that act like garbage collectors and recyclers. If any of these systems are compromised, our biological terrain becomes unhealthy. We create an environment hospitable to pathogens. Interesting to note that many herbal remedies are indeed weeds, thus collecting the body's garbage (detox) when consumed, which is part of the reason why they are historically considered medicine.

***The Lake*** — Another simple analogy is the Lake analogy. The largest element of the human body's biological terrain is water. So it helps to visualize the biological terrain as a lake. So in essence, we are a big enclosed by skin - lake. This lake of water, considered by Dr. Robert Greenberg who has a Ph.D. in Biochemistry, Doctor of Chiropractic, and a licensed Naturopathic Physician, is considered the "terrain of tomorrow". He even classifies the body's water into 3 kinds of fluids that are extracellular. They are: Intra-ocular, Cerebrospinal Fluid, and Interstitial. But for the purpose of discussion let's keep it simple, we are mostly water..

Further into our Lake analogy, our body is also comprised of roughly 100 trillion cells. The cells are what give us structure and help hold the lake together. These cells are very dependent on the condition of the lake. Now think of these 100 trillion cells, in a lake, with water outside the cells and inside the cells (interstitial). Another visual is fishing bobbers (cells) floating everywhere in the lake. If the lake's pH becomes too acid or alkaline the health of the lake is severely impacted. So too is the health of roughly 100 trillion cells. This can also happen in isolated areas of the lake (i.e. vaginal canal).

As mentioned, human bodies (the lake analogy) depend upon proper pH levels. They also depend on lessened oxidation levels and proper mineral/electrolyte balance to be optimal. The health of our cells does indeed depend upon the biological environment in and around our cells. The most valuable aspect here is pH (potential of Hydrogen). The theory is to keep all the fluids of the whole body adjusted and moving, much as a clean flowing river. That way the body can sweep things out and transfer things in. This has of course a positive impact on all cellular function itself. By analogy, keeping the lake healthy or the top soil at optimum is true prevention. The biological terrain, when in balance, tends to become inhospitable to pathogens.

We know from biology that pathogens and even cancer will create its own environment to favor itself. Why invite them in to stay or morph with a less favorable environment to begin with?

***The Vitalists*** — So is this concept of biological terrain new? A group of scientists known as vitalists were early pioneers to this terrain concept and theory. They included well-known members such as Glavani, Mesmer, and Hahnemann, who championed and favored a new paradigm shift in their day of homeostasis or balance versus simple monomorphism.

Biological Terrain is not a new science by any means. Claude Bernard, a physiologist who lived be-tween 1813-1878, shared with Louis Pasteur that he and others were missing something called the "Milieu Interior". Today, this Milieu Interior is now known as the Biological Terrain. He argued that this is what represents the environment of the cell. It determines the function and efficiency of the cell and therefore the entire organism. This also creates a less favorable home for infection too.

In July of 1962 another "vitalist", Professor Louis Claude Vincent, redefined three primary factors which are the magnetic factor, electrical factor, and di-electrical factor. In the first, a proton carries a positive magnetic field with it. This field is sensitive to alteration in what is known as Schumann's waves. The second, polarization and depolarization, are the activities of the cell and relate to oxidation and reduction of the movement of electrons.

Lastly, the dielectric represents the electrical volume through which the electrical concentration can be measured. He went on to prove biologically pure water created a pristine terrain, while unhealthy water created a sick or deadly terrain. He basically proved contaminated water could cause cancer is certain areas of France. This led to more understanding of what it means to manage the biological terrain.

***HPV Terrain*** — How does this biological terrain concept pertain to HPV and cervical cancer? The vaginal biological terrain is naturally acidic or of a low pH ($< 4.5$). It is the main mechanism controlling the populations of vaginal flora. Lactobacillus (over 20 different species), are the primary colonizing bacteria in a healthy vagina (66). Low acidity is helpful here for being detrimental to foreign pathogens entering and thriving in the vaginal canal. These lactobacilli produce hydrogen peroxide (H2O2), bacteriocins, and organic (lactic) acids, to help inactivate HIV-1, HSV-2, and other organisms. If the terrain of the vaginal canal is disrupted or Lactobacilli growth is diminished, low levels of H2O2, acids, and bacteriocins are produced. This will invite pathogens to inhabit the area (67). The biological terrain has been disturbed and is more favorable to a pathogen like HPV. The healthy populations of the vaginal canal include aerobic and anaerobic species. The point is biological terrain re-establishment is part of the holistic protocol for improving favorable outcome of HPV infection. Hormones such as estrogen and menstruation cycles are also clues to pay attention to in regards to proper vaginal terrain.

If you get serious about balancing biological terrain, not just vaginally, but all over (more quantum in nature), then changing your lifestyle, reducing stress (emotions), will provide a higher degree of success with any protocol. In the case of HPV not only will one see improved Pap test results, but a lifelong health for the rest of the body and expanded disease prevention as well.

Dr. Max Gerson who is in the Orthomolecular Medicine Hall of Fame in Ottawa Canada said it best, "Stay close to nature and its eternal laws will protect you".

# Chapter 11:
# EPIGENOMICS (Epigenetics)

"Let the body know, let the body comprehend that it is being chosen as a channel for the expression of divinity into materiality!" - Edgar Cayce (68)

***Influence and Epigenomics*** — Clean air, clean water, a vegetarian diet, restful sleep, quality supplements, exercising, detoxification, and stress reduction. Chiropractic care, acupuncture, massage, reflexology, colon hydrotherapy, Rife therapy and so many others, were at one time or are still considered, alternative. Yet an emerging science concept known as Epigenomics or epigenetics is now helping prove these are not alternative therapies, but necessary therapies!

Since the industrial revolution, man as a species, has made a great many errors. It is how we by our own nature tend to over consume, mass produce, and make waste that has contributed greatly in depleting us. This behavior has helped contribute to a whole new plethora of diseases and even superbugs. Advancements such as pursuing genetically modified organisms, creation and overuse of harsh chemicals everywhere, fluorocarbons which thin the ozone layer, and as a result help destroy the very water and air we depend on. We are only beginning to understand the kind of influence this is having on our health. It will be up to each and every one of us to take responsibility to clean up the mess, but to also understand just how this impacts our own health. We cannot simply ignore this type of impact or just leave our health challenges up to allopathic treatments, which are more chemically based. We all must take responsibility for our own health and find ways to change our own wrong doing.

For example the Journal of American Medicine (JAMA) printed an article outlining this new understanding. It stated that "90% of all illness is caused by lifestyle, the environment, stress and genetics". It went on to state that only 10% of a patient's health outcome can be directly affected by a physician or hospital. So, in a sense, 90% of all illness and recovery is up to the individual (69)! When you consider the astronomical cost of today's health care, that's not much of a return on only the 10% they can affect (by their own admission). We must still respect the emergency care we have but participate more fully in recovery and prevention of the majority of diseases.

A new science that is emerging, and that fits into the HPV protocol, is called Epigenomics. It is a science that will be part of the future of medicine. We no longer can just sit back and wait till we are sick before we seek healthcare. Not if 90% of the cause and outcome is our own doing and responsibility. This is a Quantum "leap" in health care understanding. It is a big part of what is wrong with the current medical system. It is also a Quantum "leap" in understanding what is meant by "genetics" alone.

Epi-genomics is: the inherited changes in phenotype (appearance) or gene expression caused by mechanisms other than changes in the underlying DNA sequence. In other words, human beings control their genomes by their decisions and actions, rather than they being controlled by their genes solely (remember the argument of random genetic mutations?).

It is now known that genetic influence takes place every second of everyday within an epigenome. An epigenome (above a gene) influences how a gene (genome) expresses itself. Meaning, every decision you make, impacts your genetic variables. Examples of this are thoughts (hopefully positive), what kind of sand which to eat, what you drink, even choosing to or not choosing to express an emotion, can have an influence on your genes.

Epigenetics is similar to a light switch. If a switch is turned "on", the genome will then activate or express itself. If the gene then expresses itself in a negative or incorrect way (DNA alteration or damage) things like mutagenesis take place. So we can have a gene lying dormant in our DNA, but it doesn't activate until the "switch" turns it on. In essence "we earn or even create disease" by turning on these epigenome switches. An example that this is a real science is identical twins. One may have a disease like Multiple Sclerosis and the other twin does not. Yet they have identical genomes. The one with the disease must have turned on the switch (lifestyle, stress, or environment) that activated a corrupted gene to begin with. The other twin has not influenced the switch…yet. Like the JAMA article stipulates, 90% of all disease is affected by our lifestyle, stress, environment, and genetics.

So in theory, if our genes can be influenced by lifestyle, environment, or stress, could they also be turned off, repaired, or reversed, as well? My father might say yes. Research is being done daily on epigenetics as a solution to disease. A process known as "applied intentional epigenetics" is showing promise in reversal of Autism, regardless of genetic make-up (70).

***The Evidence is in…Me!*** — I was born with something called "absence of immunoglobulin A (IGA)". As a child I was always sick. Allergies, flus, ear infections, tonsillitis, and so forth were my norm. I have a 5th grade report card showing I missed 53 days of school due to illness (glad I had good grades). I have had ear tubes put in three times, had my appendix removed, tonsils and adenoids removed, subjected to allergy desensitization injections (prescribed from scratch tests) twice a week for fourteen years. I was allergic to 270 out of 300 foods tested. The world became my enemy. I lived on antibiotics, decongestants, and antihistamines.

When I was 22 (1982) I decided to take matters into my own hands, since my parents were just following doctor's orders, I felt this was getting me nowhere.

I visited a brand new immunologist, Dr. Burr, in Appleton, Wisconsin. He politely looked at my mammoth medical history file and said this; "The problem is no one knows what the cause is. It looks like everyone (M.D.) is just treating your symptoms. We need to know what the cause is". After picking my chin off the table, it became clear to me. This is known as an "Aha" moment. It is an example of Quantum fundamental creativity thinking. I then asked "so what is the cause"? This was a new concept to me, to treat the cause, not the symptoms. He said "I don't know, but have you ever had your immunoglobulins tested"? Being in premed, I had to think hard about what that even meant. I said "no".

After the diagnosis, by blood sampling all of my immunoglobulins, the "A" immunoglobulin tested absent. The lab test showed absolute zero. He stated "This is genetic. You were born that way". So like anyone paying for advice, I asked "what I can I do?" He stated "Take vitamin C or drink lots of Orange Juice, and move to Florida. The air is better".

"How much Vitamin C is enough?" I asked. His reply (part of the reason why I even began studying integrative medicine in the first place) was "You can't take enough!" So I became a vitamin C expert. Linus Pauling (discover and Nobel prize winner on Vitamin C) became my mentor. It helped change my life. It changed my health.

The labs from Appleton Medical Center in 1982 showed my immunoglobulin "A" to be absolute zero. I still have the original test in a frame. Now, if the science of epigenomics is known to change genes for the worse, why not the better?

In 1992, after years of improving my diet (lifestyle) and supplementing with complete sources of Vitamin C, cleansing my body of toxins (environment) and using flower therapy for emotional and vital morphogenetic chakra enhancement (stress), I had a follow up lab test with Dr. Burr. The results showed my immunoglobulin "A" was now 2,200 (normal). I asked Dr. Burr "have you ever seen someone go from congenital absence of immunoglobulin A, to normal before?" He said "No, it must have been misdiagnosed". That sounded familiar.

He wouldn't even admit after 10 years, that he was the one who found it (why I framed it). How could this have happened? Was it a mis-diagnosis? The lab tests showed physical proof that it was not. This led me to explore the science of epigenetics. Could congenital anomalies be reversed? I am sure what was passed on to me was genetic. Could the sins of the father/mother be passed on, but later cured? Well, from my experience, yes. So let's explore this deeper.

***Epigenetics: Front and Center*** — As in all naturopathy, holistic, alternative, complimentary, integrative, or quantum medicine approaches, epigenetics is front and center in these fields of study. Most naturopaths just describe it differently. Epigenetics is simply a change in gene activity or expression, but not involving just 'the true genetic code'. The Human Genome project itself has a long way to go.

However, we now have discovered that the epigenome (influence or marker) on the gene itself can get passed on down. Sometimes, the influence can happen immediately to an individual's genome. Either way, the influence can be passed on. That makes it a much more interesting science.

An epigenome tends to sit on top of a gene itself. It is by comparison, much larger in size. It is energetic in nature. It is also known as a marker. A size analogy is that a gene or genome is similar in size to the planet Earth. The Epigenome by comparison in size and influence, would be like the size of the Sun. It may take us a hundred years to know what is all inside an epigenome! It already took 10 years and billions of dollars to just map the human genome itself (Earth size). But, because of emerging science like epigenetics, we definitely have found out that genes can be influenced by every single decision one makes in a day.

Again, the epigenome (marker) instructs a gene below it. To turn itself "on or off" (express itself). In other words an epigenome can influence genes to lie dormant or to activate.

This concept helps explain what is meant by genetic predisposition. We can be "pre-disposed" to a disease (i.e. Alzheimer's, Diabetes, Cancer, etc.) genetically, but it takes the epigenome influence to turn that gene "on" or express itself. Like the JAMA article shows us, every decision, choice, ingestion, toxin, thought, or action, can result in pre disposition to full blown expression. Even what we did last night, is not only affecting our gene expressions, but can even be passed on to the next generation. You may even pre-dispose your children by your lifestyle, exposure to environmental toxins, and stress, before they are ever even conceived.

During the 1980's, Dr. Lars Olov Bygren proved in Stockholm that: "conditions in the womb can affect your health, not only when you were a fetus, but well into adulthood." In 1986 Lancet Journal reported "if a pregnant woman ate poorly, her child is at a higher risk for cardiovascular disease as an adult!"

2001 Dutch journals (Acta Biotheoretica) showed the same thing. Food abuse by a single individual (mother or father) could result in just one year, producing children who died an average of 6 years earlier. Conclusion: A single season of over-eating, even as a youngster, creates a biological chain of events that lead to grandchildren dying "decades" earlier than their peers.

In 2003, Mice fed GMO (genetically modified) soy had changes in their testicles which suggests possible problems in the sperm cells. The young embryo offspring of mice that were fed GMO soy had changes in DNA expression compared to those whose parents were fed non-GMO natural soy (71).

With rats, whose mothers were fed GMO soy, 56% of the offspring died within 3 weeks compared to 9% of those whose mothers ate non-GMO soy. This is the same GMO soy that's planted in 89% of the soy fields in the U.S. supply. The only human feeding study ever conducted and published showed that genes that were inserted into soybeans (to cause them to be herbicide tolerant) transferred into human gut bacteria and was integrated stably into the DNA. This means that long after you stop eating a genetically engineered food, your own gut bacteria may be producing these foreign proteins. In general, the FDA allowed the products anyway without this type of testing because it was declared that it was "generally recognized as safe (GRAS)."

***Sins of the Father*** — The European Journal of Human Genetics (2006) studied 166 fathers who started smoking before age 11. This created a fertile ground for epigenetic changes. This study showed sons were at higher risk of obesity, CVD (cardio-vascular disease), and resulted in shorter life span of the offspring (72). So you can influence epigenetics, even when you make a dumb decision at age 10. This is not only a medical mistake by not addressing epigenetics, but a catastrophic one (passed on) because we now know all choices can affect our phenotypes.

There are 210 cell types in the human body (that we know of so far). Likely, they all have different epigenomes as well. Again, the Human Genome Project found 25,000 different genes in just 1 genome (at a cost of $3 billion). The epigenome numbers could be so many in numbers; it would create an algorithm mathematical thesis taking decades in itself to calculate.

As in the HPV holistic and quantum protocol using silver sol, changing our lifestyle choices, decreasing the amount of toxins from our environments, and managing stress, will all lead to better epigenetic influence(s). Also of course, better health information (epigenome) being passed on to the next generation. Not only does this help the outcome of the protocol for a woman with HPV in the present, but it will help the next generations too.

# Chapter 12: HOLISTIC EPIGENETIC INFLUENCE

Holistic epigenetic influence is similar to a concept known as "the pillars of health". We will outline a positive holistic epigenetic influence for HPV infection and cervical cancer.

What is the most important nutrient to the human body that you will notice very quickly if it's missing?

***Air*** — of course! How long do think you can last without it? You need this critical ingredient way more than water and food (in order of importance). More to the point, most of us will spend 90% of our life indoors during a lifetime. So it stands to reason, having fresh air is important to our health, terrain, and epigenetic influence.

The CDC recommends a HEPA filter in buildings and homes to help remove bacteria and virus from the work/home area where you spend that time. Also air sanitizers which use UV light and silver nano-particle technology are helpful indoors. I often recommend this idea before even talking about diet or water. Aromatherapy and plants also are ideal in air quality which helps balance pH in the body as well. Whatever measures we can take in a positive direction to assist our bodies with its environment, lifestyle, or stress reduction, can help reduce a negative epigenetic influence.

***Water*** — We have already discussed water a bit (structured) in the chapter on Advancement of Silver Sol Technology. But this element which is critical to life and to our daily planet doesn't always get the scrutiny it deserves. Just having clean water and plenty of it is critical to maintaining health and helping to heal in general.

Dehydration is the most discussed aspect of water with good reason. So consider this, when you are usually hungry, it may mean you are most likely thirsty. Try drinking a glass of filtered water one half hour before you eat food. If you are no longer hungry in a half hour, you were thirsty. You may not even need to eat. This contributes to better weight management.

The aspect of water that doesn't get enough attention paid to it is quality. Tap water from municipality or wells can be toxic and have an acidic pH. Even little blue plastic bottles of water you paid for from a gas station, won't mean it is a pure source of water. The water industry is largely unregulated. Use of a carbon-block filter, or an ionizer, electrolysis, reverse-osmosis, or a distiller, can be a lifesaving and sound investment.

Water in general is a powerful cleanser of poisons in the body as well as a hydrator. A good analogy is one cannot do dirty dishes with dirty water. The EPA in 2002 did a landmark study called the National Recommended Water Quality Criteria. It concluded that they found over 96,000 different poisons, carcinogens, and toxins in the nation's drinking water supplies. That study also the showed the same results of toxins were found regardless if it was well water or municipal water. In 2014, The Silent Spring Institute and the Harvard School of Public Health released results of a study, entitled, "Biomarkers for Suspected Breast Carcinogens." In it, many toxic chemicals were identified in tap water that we should avoid for breast cancer prevention. What was their recommendation? "Do not drink tap water." In order for optimal health, and less influence on epi-genomes, focus on a water filtration systems for health improvement.

***Environment*** — Take a minute to think about the environment. It is everything you are surrounded by and enveloped in. From your toxic dry cleaning gases to mercury oxide from plastics in your new car and everything else. The world is a toxic place. Even invisible radiation and electromagnetic frequency's abound. Our bodies are inundated with free radicals and our food supply doesn't keep up with all the additional chemicals we have to contend with. This was also discussed in detail in biological terrain. Maintaining a clean environment in and around you is optimal to preventing disease. Or the opposite which is creating an internal environment favorable of pathogens like HPV.

***Stress*** — Stress can be good or bad. There is healthy stress like a newborn baby or a wedding. Then there is unhealthy stress like the death of a spouse, divorce, disability, toxic friends, work, the news, multitasking, etc.

As noted by the Father of stress study Dr. Hans Selye, M.D., (Canadian Medical Hall of Fame), "Eventually chronic stress depletes the body's resources and its ability to adapt. If stress continues and remains unattended for a long period, coping functions will be compromised and illness will result."

Sleep deprivation, anxiety disorders, even hypertension, are all influenced by unaddressed stress. Anxiety alone costs the U.S. more than $42 billion in health care costs according to www.cdc.gov/mentalhealth/basics/burden.htm.

Stress reduction techniques, yoga, massage, reflexology, and flower therapy, are just a few powerful adjuncts to keep our stress levels under control and the immune system strong. This is another adjunct to creating a holistic epigenetic influence.

***Exercise*** — Exercise can be thought of in two ways, fast and slow. Fast exercise is obvious physical activity. Slow (like yoga), is more energetic and working with the subtle bodies. Both are important.

First let's touch on fast exercise. According to Dr. Gordon Pederson's dissertation research, exercise/nutrition and the combination of both helped in preventing viral infections. Regular fast exercise resulted in a 16% increase in immune cells.

He also measured an 18% increase (in NK cells) due to herbal supplementation. However, when a person exercised and took supplementation at the same time, there was a 255% increase in NK cells (17).

Second, slow exercise, is movement such as yoga, tai chi, and qi gong. It results in better balance and energetic renewal. Use of this type of exercise is on the rise. According to National Health Statistics Report for Feb. 10, 2015 issue number 79: states these modalities were 5.8% of the population in 2002. It is 10.1% in 2012. Yoga accounts for about 80% of this increase over the decade. Are you doing fast and slow exercise?

***Supplements*** — US Public Law 103-417 states: "The use of nutritional dietary supplements prevents disease, promotes wellness, and reduces long term health costs. They are safe and increase longevity and quality of life".

The supplements recommended for HPV infection and cervical cancer, are outlined in a later chapter. In general supplements are an integral part of holistic health.

***Diet*** — U.S. Dept. of Agriculture reports 92% of Americans do not get sufficient nutrients from the food they eat (73). Too much of it is over processed, over cooked, denatured, and simply dead food with added preservatives. Switching to a mostly vegetarian diet will take effort and will power, but can pay big dividends to restoring the biological terrain. Supplementing with meal replacements using green super foods is another great way to start. Many people first coming into a more holistic diet modification cannot simply change everything they are used to eating overnight. The taste buds have been conditioned since birth on what is known as S.A.D. (Standard American Diet). The typical SAD is mostly comprised of table salt, refined sugar, bad fats, simple processed carbohydrates, gluten, MSG, etc. and are over abundantly contained in the food supply. Even food manufacturers have spent tons of money trying to find the "bliss" point in food tastes to hook us on their processed foods without our knowledge. To obtain an adequate (not even considering optimal) supply of phyto-chemicals, antioxidants, vitamins, minerals, essential fatty acids, it is next to impossible to get from the denatured packaged and processed foods of today.

If you do consume meat, do so in moderation and only eat organic/grass fed when possible. Meats or red meats tend to be high in glutamine which acts as a nitrogen shuttle in the blood. This helps bring nitrogen to cancerous cells, which help make more cancerous cells.

Since cancer cells require fermentation as a metabolic process they also consume about 8 times more glucose than normal cells. It stands to reason that excess refined and processed sugars will help feed cancer cells. For example an oncogene called MicroRNA-21 that is up regulated in a variety of cancers which increases cancer growth, is stimulated by a high processed and refined sugar diet (74).

Don Ayer, Ph.D., a Huntsman Cancer Institute investigator and professor in the Dept. of Oncological Sciences at the University of Utah discovered that by restricting glutamine availability, glucose was not well utilized by cancer cells. They became short circuited. His research helped show glutamine and sugar are inter-dependent. So reduction in red meats and excess sugar is a diet consideration in cervical cancer management.

Researchers at the University of Virginia in British Columbia followed 200 people who had "spontaneous remission of cancer". In all, 87% of those people had switched to a more vegetarian diet (75).

Mediterranean-type diets also have merit here. It helps to keep your body in better balance of omega-3, 5, 6, 7, and 9's. The odd number omegas are what the body desires. The S.A.D. diet tends to contain up to 30 times more omega-6 fats than 3's. Even sourcing your olive oils requires research as most oils sold commercially today are adulterated.

It takes time to learn to prepare "live" foods and time to change over to more vegetarian lifestyle. All this greatly enhances the biological terrain more favorably and promote pleomorphism ideals.

***Vibrational Medicine and Vital Energy*** — Dr. Yury Kronn, a major contributor to the field of non-linear quantum radio-physics once said, "Only 10% of the energy in the universe is measurable. That leaves 9 times as much subtle forms of energy that we can draw from (76)." It is these subtle energy forms that we are addressing with a holistic quantum approach. One application is the chakras of the human body. In particular with HPV infection, we are most concerned with the second chakra. This 2nd chakra is one of many morphogenetic fields that help process vibrational energy of specific frequencies or vital energy. This chakra is centered on the vibrational energy of family, sex, money, and even power. The organs associated with this chakra do contain the uterus/cervix. So by helping balance vital energy in this chakra, it helps ensure organs and tissues are regenerated from past and current insults. Also it reduces influence of a negative nature to these organ areas.

In 1928 Edgar Cayce (the sleeping prophet) channeled this; "The human body is made up of electronic vibrations, with each atom and element of the body, each organ and organism, having its electronic unit of vibration necessary for the sustenance of, and equilibrium in, that particular organism." He went on to say that by injury or by disease, internal or external, elements of the body become deficient in energy and can no longer reproduce (cells) or sustain (77).

Quantum physics helps us understand that human beings are more than single dimensional beings. We are multi-dimensional. The physical body is what we see in the mirror and are acutely aware of all the time. It is also the densest. Other dimensional fields do exist such as the vital energy body, the mental, supra-mental, and bliss body. In 1981, R. Sheldrake helped prove that nonphysical vital energy (morphogenetic) fields are necessary to help create our physical body. All of the latter of these "other dimensional fields" are of higher vibration and much more subtle. Jung's typology (2004) gave a simpler idea: the physical body is where we 'sense'. Further, the vital body is where we 'feel', the mental is where we 'think', the supra-mental is the house of 'intellect', and the bliss is 'limitless joy or the soul'.

Each of these subtle bodies is then connected to the physical body by energy itself (chakra points or wheels). It is similar to a network of sorts. Subtle energy can come into and even out of the physical body through these fields by using chakras, which are in essence portals and transformers of energy. These portals help process frequencies into biological manifestations.

The endocrine system is the most physical part connected (energetically) to these chakras. The chakras can be thought to assist in blueprints of manifestation. Chakras are able to affect mood, behavior, hormonal influence, and the cellular matrix. Again, the chakra we want to help influence in a positive way here for HPV infection is the "sacral" chakra or 2nd chakra. It is a part of a known line of seven that follow ascendingly up the spine from the coccyx area to the top of the cranium (78).

The chakras help play a vital role in consciousness itself. They have special regard to emotional states. If the chakras are properly balanced, they help maintain homeostasis. Abnormal function can create weakness in the associated area of the physical body. Chakras provide a type of vital or nutritive subtle energy for the physical.

The second chakra is known by many names such as the navel, gonadal, splenic, or sacral chakra. It is considered the seat of sexuality. It is associated with the gonads, reproductive organs, urinary bladder, and intestines. Symbolically it is linked with the element of water. Given this background, the importance of chakra balancing to cervical cancer is tantamount in the holistic quantum approach.

A virus, like HPV, may be vibrationally linked to an area of weakness. If a virus enters the vaginal canal, and the second chakra is weak from a stressor, this can be an influencer for certain infection to take hold. As in the common cold, one tends to earn the cold, not catch it.

There are many protocols for dealing with an imbalanced chakra. A few are color therapy; homeopathy, flower therapy, energy massage, counseling, etc.

# Chapter 13: THE PROTOCOL

**Silver sol gel (24ppm)** in a 3 oz. tube (manufactured by the same supplier for all participants marketed as Silver Shield). The gel is squeezed from the tube, an applied in the amount resembling a U.S. nickel in size. This is applied or dabbed onto the tip of a vaginal insert tampon (see list in Case studies).

The tampon insert itself is preferred to be non-bleached, if can be obtained that way. The nickel sized gob of silver sol gel is put on the end of that tampon and inserted vaginally. Participants were instructed to keep the tampon with silver sol gel in place, inside the vagina, for at least 60 minutes. Studies of silver sol show contact time is generally 10-12 minutes, but it was felt for proper contact inside the vagina to help reach the cervix area, to use 60 minutes due to body movements. Many women left it in longer which was not necessary, but easier on their lifestyle. It was also advised it could be inserted at night time and taken out in the a.m. The only stipulation was contact time had to be a minimum of 12 minutes. The silver sol gel and tampon application is the main protocol ingredient.

You can also do this silver sol insertion in multiple time frames. Such as inserting a tampon coated with silver sol gel for 30 minutes a day, 3 - 4 times a day. Most women opted for 1 time a day. But if changing out tampons due to menstruation, the point is mute. It was necessary that the tampon insertion was done for a minimum of seven days or nights in a row. They were all instructed not to forget this part: daily application for 7 days/nights up to 60 minutes at an insert.

The Silver sol gel used in study is a Class I medical device approved by the FDA. It is marketed as a "wound dressing gel". It contains a proprietary silver sol concentration of 24 ppm (nano-silver at .o1 micron) in a 3 oz. tube of purified water and a carbomer. This is a water–based hydro gel for use in a moist wound care management as well. The gel has been evaluated in standard tests that show it can reduce the levels of common microorganisms including Staphylococcus aureus, Pseudomonas aeruginosa, Escherichia coli, Methicillin Resistant Staphylococcus Aureus (MRSA), and VRE, as well as fungi such as Candida albicans and Aspergillus Niger (79).

As a side consideration, one can also pump two – three ounces of liquid silver sol in a douche form, inter-vaginally. The gel method is preferred due to the ability of the gel to "stick" ensuring contact time. Only silver sol gel was used in all case studies. But if using the liquid (gel not available), then mix two ounces of silver sol liquid (minimum 20ppm) with two-three ounces of distilled water. Hold it in place vaginally (not ideal) for 15 minutes to ensure contact time. This is only noted as it can be done in conjunction with the gel or as a "cleanse" of the vaginal area in general.

Another side note: Liquid or gel can be used in a panty liner for an added benefit. Also used in the bath tub by adding in 4 ounces of silver to the water and soaking for about 25 minutes. This will help "cleanse" the anogenital regions.

# Chapter 14:
# ADDITIONAL OPTIONS WITH SILVER SOL GEL PROTOCOL

***Immune Discussion*** — Keeping the immune system strong can also help clear out HPV on its own. All techniques that enhance the immune system hold promise. Anything that may damage the immune system is not. Supporting or modulating the immune system simply improves ones physiology. The immune systems job is to destroy foreign invaders and is separated into two systems the Th1 and Th2 response. For purpose of discussion the Th1 response is like the first team on the scene. If an HPV virus is strong enough to outlast the Th1 team, then the Th2 team kicks in. The Th2 team helps create antibodies against that virus, so white blood cells can finish the virus off (80).

Hippocrates said "healing is a matter of time, but it is sometimes a matter of opportunity." As is the case with any dis-ease, it is a matter of time and opportunity. We need to keep in mind we need time to heal, because none of us with chronic conditions really get sick overnight. It takes time to tip the scales in favor of a pathogen. It takes time to tip the scales back to balance. It has been my experience those who look for a quantum holistic approach, are usually ready for it. Many of my clients have commented over the years "I am sick and tired of being sick and tired". Allopathic treatment often only offers drugs and surgery and it has led them to a new approach.

The immune system in HPV infection requires strengthening and support to naturally overcome this pathogen. Combined with a silver aqua sol gel, this is a very powerful course. The immune system is designed to do one thing - kill things. This design is to 'turn on' against bio-toxins (bacteria, virus, parasites, etc.). Also, the immune system assists in the cleaning up of old cells necessary for cancer to NOT develop in the first place. Normally, a virus attempts to hide from the immune system by infiltrating a cell. The cell gives off a marker on the cell membrane to alert this system that it has been invaded. Through phagocytosis, immune killer cells (see below) engulf the entire cell containing the virus and kill both the cell and pathogen virus in the process.

The part of the immune system that is important here is components of blood that help the body fight infections and other diseases. White blood cells can be categorized as either granulocytes or mononuclear leukocytes. Mononuclear leukocytes are further sub-grouped into monocytes and lymphocytes. Lymphocytes, found in the blood, tissues and lymphoid organs (i.e. spleen), attack antigens (foreign). The main lymphocyte sub-types are B-cells, T-cells, and natural killer (NK) cells. B-cells make antibodies that are stimulated by infection.

Lymphatic massage to support the Spleen organ is also favorable. An interesting note on anatomy of the Spleen, if you were to dissect a cadaver spleen, you would find inside of it another spleen. Also ribs, two kidneys, a pancreas, stomach, diaphragm, an aorta, and a liver. The Chinese for centuries have regarded the spleen for the power of digestion, circulation, blood quality, and immunity.

***Vitamin D3*** — Research has suggested and pointed out the value of Vitamin D3 supplementation in various types of cancers such as colon and breast. It is even been suggested for all cancers. The Vall d 'Hebron Institute of Oncology (VHIO), in collaboration with the Alberto Sols Institute of Biomedical Research (CSIC-UAB), demonstrated the powerful role of Vitamin D. The results published in the journal PLoS One, showed a slowdown in the action of a key protein in the transformation process of colon cancer cells. Their supposition was that Vitamin D is essential in the prevention and treatment of colon cancer, and all cancers for that matter.

In March of 2009 the Archives of Internal Medicine noted that supplementing just 1,000 IU/d's a day of Vitamin D3 showed a 40% reduction in colds and flu. It was even was on par as being more effective than a flu shot. This demonstrates an integrated approach to viral prevention and cancer development helping to positively influence the biological terrain.

Vitamin D deficiency is seen more readily in colder climates but is also depleted due to sunscreen promotion in warm climates too. We can help our body obtain some Vitamin D from good oils and raw milk consumption but the body mostly manufactures it from exposure to sunlight, converting sunlight to vitamin D from our cholesterol. The body uses cholesterol to convert it to Vitamin D3 in the skin in as little as twenty minutes, twice a week sun exposure. Due to sun blockers and low cholesterol prescriptions, could low levels be contributing to increases in cancer? Therefore, it is advised in this protocol to consider Vitamin D3 supplementation as an option. Vitamin D2 (man-made) is discouraged and is considered synthetic.

Currently the Institute of Medicine (IOM) and with guidance of 'Health Canada' provides national supplement advice for the people of Canada and the United States. For years scientists have postulated that Vitamin D levels for optimum health need to be much higher that currently recommended. The IOM is now advocating an RDA of 4,000 to 10,000 IU/d, Body Mass Index dependent. The IOM is even going so far as to propose upper limits of 20,000 IU/d (81).

***pH balancing*** — Alkalizing the body with proper foods and minerals is an essential part of the protocol for many health reasons. Assisting the body with being more alkaline (as most people are acidic) helps with elimination of toxic substances. In turn, it helps support bones, joints, and oxygenation. If not, acidity or acidosis takes place most notably in the saliva and urine. The Standard American Diet (S.A.D. diet) is heavily acid. As mentioned previously, this is important in balancing biological terrain and epigenetic positive influence. Hippocrates himself even suggested an alkaline diet.

Focusing on an 80% alkaline diet includes lots of vegetables, green juices, and tropical fruits. It is best to avoid red meats, processed and refined sugars, dairy, soda, white foods and flours, and artificial sweeteners. As discussed previously with glutamine and sugar connections. Prescriptions, white vinegar, liquor, coffee, tobacco are just some of the other offenders. Other factors that contribute to a poor pH balance are unresolved stress, negative emotions, bad food combining (no proteins with starch), not chewing your food completely, lack of exercise, and insufficient enzyme production in the gut.

Instructions were given, although voluntary to alkalize drinking water by using 1 tsp. baking soda to a 12 oz. glass of water per day. Lemons are also very alkalizing. Liquid Chlorophyll could also be added to water.

Testing pH was not necessary but if they decided to do this it was suggested to be done in the home with pH test strips for saliva and urine. It was suggested to test first thing in a.m. with urine and saliva before eating. Then, obtain an average over a couple of days for the base line of these bodily fluids. Most strips are available in pharmacies or online and come with a color card for evaluation.

***Antioxidants*** — It is suggested to take proanthocyanidins (polyphenols) or doses of antioxidants like vitamin C in general, which helps with the scavenging of cell-damaging free radicals. There may be slight oxidation from the carbomers of silver sol gel ph. Free radicals are reactive molecules that can damage DNA. Proanthocyanidins are known to increase the number and activity of white blood cells. This also helps to neutralize the free radicals from pathogens and offset acidity issues from oxidation in the vagina.

Viruses are also a known cause of oxidation. They produce an increased load of free radicals inside cells that are infected. This in turn can produce what is known as slime layer around the infected cells to ward off the immune system response attack. So the protocol calls for optional antioxidants. Not just any antioxidant but antioxidants that also are called pro-oxidant. Curcumin, green tea, vitamin C, are examples of an antioxidant and pro-oxidant. Pro-oxidant components actually cause free radical increase (in this case a good thing) inside a cancer cell, causing eventual death of the infected cancer cell, similar to chemotherapy. Certain antioxidants (like proanthocyanidins), even inhibit certain enzymes that stop abnormal apoptosis.

The source used here is a blend of proanthocyanidins from grape seed and maritime pine bark. The blend is standardized. The dose used is 60 mg four times a day for a week. Then 60 mg two time a day for up to three months. The goal is not overdose antioxidants but assist the body in balance. If using vitamin C antioxidant make sure it is a whole form vitamin and not a chemical isolate. Then this is only a fraction of the whole. For example, vitamin C must contain rutin, citrus bioflavonoids, hesperidin, rose hips, and/or other components such as Factor K, J, P, and Tyrosinase. In its whole form of vitamin C it is alkalizing and not acidic. Most over the counter Vitamin C's are just plain ascorbic acid which is acifying.

The vagina has a rough pH of 5.9. Silver sol used in this protocol is roughly a pH of 4.5. So oxidation does take place and to counter that, an antioxidant of grape seed and pine bark was used but considered optional. Silver sol gel can tend to soften vaginal mucosa – which can pull in moisture, especially with a thinner vaginal wall due to aging. So addressing oxidation is a concern.

Debate has taken place recently about the use of over the counter antioxidants in general. So it is worth noting here that in the case of modern oncologists suggesting the "dangers" of antioxidant therapy, they should not call the kettle black. Oncologists may prescribe Amifostine and Dexrazone in their practice. These are known prescription antioxidants. They are used in conjunction with medications such as chemotherapy and/or radiation to help decrease the side effects of chemo and radiation which produce enormous amounts of free radicals and destroy healthy surrounding tissues (82).

***Flower Therapy*** — As an adjunct to the silver sol gel protocol, holistic flower therapy is recommended. This is because of chakra (morphogenetic fields) imbalance and to help solidify the mind/body connection. This will help overcome the emotional fear of a diagnosis like cervical cancer or HPV. Just hearing the words "cervical cancer" or "cancer" in general is an emotional reaction and downright scary.

The feeling or emotion of fear for example is just that, a feeling or signal. It is always helpful to get the person back in control of that fear. After all, the individual is in control, not the emotion. The best way to address this is to acknowledge it first. To notice it is there. Get the person to realize it is ok to feel this way. This helps tell the subconscious mind that you have noticed this feeling. Sometimes it will dissolve on its own just from this ideal.

The mind/body connection is very powerful. Whatever the mind is speaking the body hears and even obeys. The body responds to what you truly think and feel. Attention to this part of us is critical in any healing process. People who tend to suppress their feelings are far more likely to develop cancer than those who express their feelings (83). So, dealing with the emotions and mind/body connection can only facilitate true healing.

If not able to express fear, balancing the chakras with flower therapy may be an option. This is a non-invasive and quantum approach to balancing the morphogenetic fields of the body. To help promote healing from powerful negative emotions that can interfere with rational decision making. Left unchecked can even influence the physical organs themselves (morphogenetic). This is especially true of the first and second chakras. Mentioned earlier, this is where the reproductive organs are located physically as well. The first chakra is involved in survival and must be properly adjusted to promote new tissues based on morphogenetic instructions to organs and cells.

Another important consideration in healing form an HPV infection, or any dis-ease for that matter, is what is known as the placebo effect. This is an example of the mind/body connection. The word "placebo" is Latin for "I shall please". It comes about when someone heals because they think they are being given an effective treatment. Many studies have proven this is a real force.

But the opposite is also true. Something called the "nocebo". It is when a person thinks they are not going to recover, so they do not. Either way, the body and mind are responding to a person's feelings and thoughts.

The choice remedy for this protocol is the Five-Flower formula, reintroduced by Dr. Edward Bach in the early part of the 20th century. This remedy deals with the emotional imbalance and energetic imbalance from fear, anxiety, panic, or disorientation. If anyone questions the efficacy of flower therapy, they may never have used it on animals. They respond beautifully to flower therapy and you can't use the power of suggestion here. No placebo or nocebo effect.

The combination of Cherry Plum, Clematis, Impatiens, Rocks Rose, and Star of Bethlehem, make up this age old homeopathic similar recipe. Used for any time of trauma or shock, as in the case of a HPV infection or cervical cancer diagnosis, it literally helps the consciousness part of us stay connected with the physical body especially due to stress. We must become proactive and positive to affect any outcome favorably.

***Eleuthro (Siberian Ginseng)*** — One of herbs that may help with HPV clearing is Eleutherococcus senticosus, A.K.A.: Siberian Ginseng or Taiga root. It is a powerful adaptogen, immune-stimulant, tonic, and alterative. This plant is substantially different than the Panax variety of Ginsengs. One of the major differences is that it can be taken by both genders for long periods of time (Hippocrates). There was a study done in East Germany and Russia in the 50's. Eleven thousand people in the study, with 14 Ph.D.'s contributing papers on the subject. Their conclusions by consensus showed that when 500 mg. of Eleuthero was consumed every day without missing a dose, those studied had 100% protection from every viral infection known to man (84).

Eleuthro was used in this protocol only once. One volunteer was already taking it and was allowed to continue usage. Since the Pap test and HPV test were positive upon entry into the protocol, it was felt it had minimal bearing on the outcome.

# Chapter 15:
# CASE STUDIES
(last names omitted for confidentiality)

***Background*** — The previous chapters have all led up to the background and understanding of how to use this quantum holistic protocol, using silver sol gel, with actual case studies. The treatments outlined below are integrative for the best outcome of the patient and to help validate the study. Follow up HPV testing and Pap was performed by a qualified medical physician. All case studies involved voluntarily using the protocol silver sol gel either in conjunction with traditional care or in lieu of.

All case study participants were instructed to consult with their conventional allopathic physicians or oncologists. All who did volunteer were instructed to get permission, or inform at least, their respective physicians.

Time was a factor (mostly based on Pap classification). Those who volunteered commented that they had months or years before the next Pap/HPV re-test was to be done on a follow up GYN exam. They were instructed that they may have to have to be persistent to get a re-test, even if out of pocket expense, within a timely frame. The time line outlined was up to three months, in case the protocol needed to be adjusted. All agreed to this for the purpose of the study since this was an integrated non-invasive safe approach.

Having a relationship with a conventional allopathic doctor was necessary for assessing progress (follow up Pap smears or HPV tests) and those tests were brought in for evaluation and follow up. The protocol discussed with each of the case studies became that case study participant's decision. Many times, the decision was without their respective physician's agreement. As all, did not want to wait months or years for a follow up test to show potential improvement. This was instrumental in the time frame outcome and how quickly those who tested positive recovered.

Again, strong emphasis was made to inform, obtain follow up Pap, and work with their conventional doctors, to give the Doctors a chance to monitor how effective this silver sol gel protocol can be. The protocol was not meant to be used as a substitute for traditional medical care. Nor was it prescriptive. No claims, guarantees, or assurances were promised other than safety of silver sol gel as a class one medical device.

In Quantum Physics we discuss the concept of non-locality. This is where thoughts and ideas can be shared by more than one person across distances but, we may not be aware others have similar ideas. Non-locality helps explain how two or more people can have same or similar creative ideas across space and time without any local contact between them. The research found others were already doing something similar in different locations but with liquid silver sols as a douche. Even in discussion with other practitioners, silver sol gel was offered intra vaginally for HPV to their respective clients but not being done in a protocol/study with actual case study participants. It was mostly offered as a suggestion in other circles.

Dr. Cynthia L. Eaton MD Fellow Amer. College of OB/GYN, American Academy of Antiaging is known to use clinical application of silver sol technology. So is Dr. Gordon Pedersen, Ph.D. in Toxicology from Utah State. He is a director of the Institute of Alternative Medicine and nominated to chair of the United States Pharmacopoeia Review Board Natural Products Committee. They both demonstrate in a DVD entitled "Silver Solutions: Women's Health" various applications that can be done with silver sol technology. This is outlined in an instructional video which shows the legitimacy of this protocol (6).

They discuss how Silver sol hits the cause and symptoms of HPV at the same time. Dr. Pedersen and Dr. Eaton recommended using silver sol in the vaginal vault, as being best way for treatment. They used a douche which is 50% silver sol and 50% distilled water. In this study protocol, the recommendation here is using silver sol gel (versus douches) for ease of application and longer contact time.

In summary, all participants were instructed to use silver sol gel on a tampon for at least seven straight days for up to 60 minutes, this was the main method and material. A checklist was given to each participant for a holistic protocol. Most used silver sol this way ongoing for months due to the efficacy. Many of the case study women commented that it proved to be an excellent vaginal lubricant upon intercourse. Silver sol gel can be used on a condom. It won't disrupt spermicides or prescriptions. It can be used after hysterectomy, again as a lubricant, for ongoing vaginal hygiene, and help assist with itching symptoms. Many of the participants noted vaginal pain/ itching lessened in as little as 24-48 hours.

All participants were given an understanding of the immune system in consultation.

***PROTOCOL LIST:*** given to each participant:

| ITEM | NEEDED |
|---|---|
| **Silver Sol Gel (24ppm)** | 1 tube (3 oz.) - dab size of nickel on end of tampon.<br>Tampon of choice, must be vaginal vault inserts. Rec. non-bleached tampon.<br>Insert daily for seven straight days, minimum of 1 hour contact time. |
| *Optional:* | |
| Vitamin D3 2,000 IU/d | 1 time a day |
| pH balancing instruction/ diet modification | Ongoing |
| Antioxidant supplement (Grape seed/Pine bark) | 60mg 4 times a day/week – 60mg 2 times a day thereafter |
| Flower Therapy | Five Flower Remedy. 8-10 drops under the tongue, in a.m. and again p.m. Nothing in mouth 15 minutes before or after administration. |

## *The 18 Female Case Study Participants:*

### Sally M. 33

Sally was recently divorced. She was seen in our clinic in October of 2013. She presented a class IIA (no obvious para-metrial involvement) Pap. The diagnosis was cervical carcinoma and was advised by her OB/GYN physician to do nothing. Just to come back for a re-check in 3 months, for additional Pap test and possible biopsy. Her physician "remarked" she may have HPV. Sally remarked she asked for further testing, which was done and did reveal positive HPV test. No medications were given and upon background consultation, she answered she had no symptoms except for some itching. Her menstruation cycles were considered normal.

Sally did not want to wait 3 months. We outlined the protocol, which was well received by her. She began with Silver sol gel administered with a tampon for seven days/60 minutes. She decided to continue administration after that at times with a vaginal applicator. She said she did this because she "felt good" doing silver sol gel, even after the seven days recommended. She was instructed to take proanthocyanidin antioxidant supplements made from maritime pine bark and grape seed of 60mg 3 x a day for month. Her diet was modified to include cruciferous vegetables with restriction on red meat, wheat flour, and dairy. Also added was a flower essence called 5 Flower or Distress Remedy developed by Dr. Bach for emotional distress from the diagnosis and due to her recent divorce. She blamed her ex for this diagnosis in her consults. So from a holistic standpoint, 2nd chakra balancing became evident to positively affect her morphogenetic field. Last, she was advised to use the silver sol gel with any sexual intercourse, but she indicated "she was through with men."

Sally's next Pap test was negative in January 2014 and she also tested negative for HPV. Her doctor remarked "she most likely cleared this on her own". She told him about the protocol and he just sighed.

She had a follow up in six months (June 2014) which produced the same test results as of January's Pap/HPV test. She has decided to continue with bi-annual Pap screens. She has had no abnormal Pap test since protocol initiation. She is still a client here and continues to use silver aqua sol gel now (with intercourse) as life would have it, she has a new man in her life.

**Janet K. 29**

Janet was referred by her sister Beth to our office for natural help with anxiety in July 8th, 2013. She is a current smoker. Her current medication was Xanax. Upon consultation here she mentioned that she had vaginal itching and odor. She was instructed to see her regular physician for potential Pap smear as she had never had a routine Pap smear in her life. She agreed to start modifying her diet to a more alkaline base and started five flower essences at night and mornings to ease anxiety naturally. Flower therapy is not contraindicated with medications.

She returned 3 months later for follow up consult for anxiety which improved with flower therapy. She has discontinued her Xanax, with her physician's permission. She did present a Pap test result showing she had a Class IIIA result. She was told by her physician she had "carcinoma in situ" or severe dysplasia. She was advised to have a conization (cryotherapy) at a later date to be determined.

She indicated that she preferred not to have this type of procedure. She was given the complimentary option of the silver sol gel protocol. Janet agreed immediately. She decided to give this a month and see her physician for consultation of cryosurgery.

She was taking a calcium supplement with Vitamin D. Was advised this is ok to continue as it is part of the protocol checklist. She also continued the five flower remedy due to her history of anxiety. She was instructed to give the protocol information to her physician.

She did not return for her scheduled appointment in a month but, called me two months later to tell me that a "bug or parasite" came out of her vaginal area during a bath. She wanted to know if the silver sol did this. I asked if she was continuing using the silver sol gel and she said "yes I do daily, I feel it has stopped any itching and odor". I instructed her that silver sol gel is anti-microbial, anti-viral, anti-fungal, and has some history of anti-parasitic properties. She asked if she should continue using the gel indefinitely. We discussed since it is not toxic to the body, yes. She also noted increased energy over the course of this time, which she felt was due to diet modification and less anxiety. I agreed. She noticed her anxiety levels were greatly diminished with food modifications, flower therapy, and felt the silver sol protocol was helping her esteem.

In November of 2013 she came into the office for a follow up consult and was extremely pleasant and excited. She had a Pap test which came back Class I. She also indicated she had no more vaginal odor or itching. She cancelled the conization on her own accord. She remarked her physician was dismayed she chose not to do the surgery but was comfortable in her test result and seemed happy for her. She continues to be seen and has quit smoking! She has referred many clients.

**Jodi L. 48**

History of client: Gravida 3, para 3. This is a woman who had relatively no health issues up until her husband was diagnosed with cancer. Shortly after this diagnosis, April 2014, she noticed she became irregular in her menstrual periods. In May of 2014, she recorded the cycle changed from "on time" every 21 days but irregular flow to "irregular" with spotting in between and about every 30 days instead. In July of 2014 she reported 36 days to a cycle with ongoing spotting. In August she noted amenorrhea (no cycle for 60 days).

She then had a visit with her gynecologist as of Aug. 8th 2014 with a diagnostic trans-vaginal ultrasound and a cervical biopsy. She had complications of those procedures and noted bleeding from the biopsy until Aug. 19th. Biopsy and Pap test Class IIA confirmed HPV infection. She had an ultrasound assessment showing endometrial hyperplasia at 15.15 mm, but considered on assessment as a normal uterus.

She was seen in our office on August 13th 2014 for natural options and we recommended the silver gel protocol which she started that day. Five flower remedy (due to her husband), antioxidants, and vitamin D3, were chosen as well.

On August 19th 2014 she called to inform us that all bleeding stopped with the gel. Since this was the seventh day of protocol she was amazed. She continued follow up with our clinic by phone and stopped the tampon insertion after a week and a half.

On September 2nd 2014 she returned for her gynecological visit and was pronounced "clear" on colposcopy with no abnormalities. She has noted normal menstrual flow and regularity returned. A follow up Pap test was also negative and negative test for HPV. She continues to follow protocol outlines and uses the silver gel for intercourse and prevention.

**Susan R. 53**

Susan entered our office and presented with an abnormal Class II Pap smear noted as "suboptimal" in April of 2010. Inflammation was also noted, possibly indicating an infection. She tested for HPV positive. She has a history of multiple sex partners and 2 past marriages. She is currently married to her third as of this time. She complained of vaginal irritation upon intercourse and a "dry" feeling. She is a menopausal female with nightly hot flashes.

She opted for the silver protocol gel as being less invasive than potential cryosurgery or even a hysterectomy as suggested by her physician. She feels her condition is not serious enough to warrant a hysterectomy. She chose to correct her diet as best she can by pH balancing. She did the silver sol protocol for seven days.

After a month she noticed no irritation and had continued using silver sol gel with intercourse. This helped with any vaginal dryness and she felt way more antiseptic than KY jelly, which she always used prior.

Her follow up Pap smear in June was clear and noted as "satisfactory." No mention of inflammation. She was pronounced by her physician as HPV clear. She is currently using a wild yam progesterone cream 25 mg for natural reduction of hot flashes, opting not to use hormone replacement therapy allopathically. Her physician commented he will follow her up again for possible hysterectomy if need be. She felt he had no clue what he was talking about.

**Cindy K. 24**

Cindy came to our office in February 8th of 2010. She was complaining of vaginal bleeding, odor, and irritation. Her Pap showed LGSIL (low grade squamous intraepithelial lesions) –cell changes caused by HPV. This is also called CIN I mild dysplasia, caused by HPV. CIN means Cervical Intraepithelial Neoplasia.

She is currently in a local college and admitted to multiple partners with unprotected intercourse. She was referred here by her mother. Upon consult she said she had been vaccinated for HPV (3 doses) in a college clinic in Wisconsin in spring of 2009. She had been taking a prescription anti-viral upon consult, but felt it best to add a holistic protocol (using the silver gel protocol) with her mother's insistence. She was instructed to use the tampon insertion for seven days. She was also advised by her physician and this clinic, to use "protective" measures such as a condom. She is currently on prescription birth control pills (BCP).

As of June 13th 2011 she is asymptomatic. She tested negative for HPV. She stated she felt the anti-viral, which was discontinued, did nothing to help her irritation and only felt relief of symptoms within a week of using the silver gel. She did no other options of the protocol, just the gel. She continues to use it going forward, applying it to condoms upon intercourse. She commented that this was a very successful approach and continues to use silver sol gel to this day.

**Austria K.** 55

Austria came to this office July 12th 2012 with a positive test 3 years ago for the HPV virus. She has had only one abnormal Pap smear in the past. She has had 2 husbands in 37 years. She indicated these were the only 2 sex partners during her life. She felt scared. She did not know which husband was the carrier of HPV in her words. She felt that one of those being uncircumcised might be the one. She felt that the foreskin could harbor virus and bacteria. She stated she was "not blaming him, for the symptoms are silent in men".

She felt bad not having a new pap smear in 3 years. This was because she lost her job and insurance and felt she could not afford additional tests. Her anxiety was very high. We spent a great deal of time discussing HPV and I referred her to the internet medical sites as well. She was encouraged to pay for a Pap test regardless. She feels this information is not being passed on to others enough as many women do not understand this problem. That is the key, education. She noted she has talked to many people and feels at least 75% do not know what HPV is. "That is scary" she remarked. "My granddaughter is going to be vaccinated if I can help it. She just turned 15 years old".

At insistence, she did have a Pap test on July 22nd 2014 that showed LGSIL (low grade squamous intraepithelial lesions) –cell changes caused by HPV, also called CIN I mild dysplasia caused by HPV.

She agreed to try the silver sol protocol as it is also cost effective. It was the least expensive option for her versus what is known as a LEEP. Her physician indicated it was an aggressive procedure. But due to her age, and since she was HPV positive 3 years ago, recommended it. A LEEP is a Loop Electrosurgical Excision Procedure.

She chose the not to do the LEEP at this time but instead try the silver sol gel protocol. She also agreed to modify her diet and use five flower therapies due to her fear noted above.

The next day she called me to ask if I drugged her, as she felt so calm. After much discussion she now realizes, this is just a side benefit of the flower therapy, which is subtle and used for fear.

She had a follow up Pap test August 26th 2014 and was considered negative for any atypical cells or HPV. She will be monitored by future Pap tests.

She still feels vaccination for her granddaughter is necessary.

**Cassandra M. 44**

Cassandra is divorcee and came here September 16th 2013. She has been in several long relationships after her divorce of five years ago. She enjoys the single life and has been very good about not taking any risks with sexual partners. She currently uses condoms.

She stated she had an abnormal Pap smear four years ago (2009) and discovered that she was infected with HPV. She had a colposcopy and was told that everything was normal after that, but was instructed that she should have a Pap smear every six months.

She had several more mildly abnormal Pap smears, and the HPV test was always positive. This was in turn followed by two normal Pap smears. She was told by her physician that the HPV must have resolved on its own.

Then 18 months ago (2012), her Pap smear at that time was interpreted as ASCUS (Atypical squamous cells of undetermined significance). She was advised that this was "nothing to worry about". She tested positive however for HPV and felt at that time that the "HPV was back". She was adamant that she had been using condoms during intercourse and couldn't understand how this virus could come back after being told it resolved. Two consequent normal Pap smears followed her "nothing to worry about" smear, but she is still positive for HPV as of September 16th 2014.

She commented that the gynecological group she always used joined a hospital system in her city this year. She had trouble getting an appointment, and the doctor she had seen for years, retired. She is now being followed up by a nurse practitioner (NP). Her NP advised her that since she had two normal pap smears in a row over the last year, she had to follow the new screening guidelines. Therefore, the tests could only be performed every two years going forward. Then if the Pap smear in two years was normal, it could only be done every three years. She feels her concerns about HPV were brushed aside when her NP stated "Everyone has this."

So Cassandra decided on the silver sol protocol versus waiting. She opted for diet modification and antioxidant supplements. We discussed options of another provider to follow her up on and for another Pap and HPV test. She was referred to a general practitioner who agreed to do the tests.

November 11th 2014 her Pap was "negative" and tested "negative" for HPV. Her new practitioner suggested two years to retest. She continues to use silver sol with condoms for prevention and takes Vitamin D3 daily.

**Cynthia A.** 25

Cynthia was referred to our office May 27th 2013 and immediately indicated she was full of fear and sleeplessness. She is divorced and has an 18 month old son. She explained her ex-husband cheated on her very regularly. It was even before the birth of her son, which she found out later. She is currently seeing "a great guy and have been with him for a year". She had been to the health department to get a prescription for birth control pills and is going back to college. A Pap test was performed and they found precancerous cells with inflammation. She was told she is HPV positive and may have cervical cancer. Further testing was suggested in a year.

She wanted to volunteer for the silver sol gel protocol. She does not wish to wait on this. She was already taking a vitamin D supplement and felt her diet was already good, as she is vegetarian. She started the silver sol protocol the next day.

Cynthia's next Pap (her own expense) on June 24th was negative and clear. The inflammation is nonexistent. Testing for HPV was also negative. She was told it probably cleared on its own even after mentioning the silver sol gel to the health department who warned her "to not fall under charlatan spells". They insisted she become vaccinated, which she has refused to do on her own accord. She felt the research and proof of vaccinations is "weak".

**Paula P. 45**

Paula entered our office for the silver sol protocol on May 13th 2011. She had always been very careful about having regular, annual GYN check-ups. So it was in December of 2010 that her doctor told her she had an irregular Pap test result. The Pap indicated precancerous cells (stage II) were present and she was HPV positive. She stated she was tested for HPV due to her age and history. She also gave a history of previous pelvic exams that she had apparently been born with a cervical lesion. The history also noted 'tendencies to have infrequent mild infection'. She was put on antibiotics three times, over a nine year span for this.

Her history included a second Pap test in February 2011, indicating cervical cancer and that it had advanced. Her Pap showed HG SIL (High grade squamous intraepithelial lesions) or moderate dysplasia CIN II. This is where abnormal cells make up ½ of the thickness surface lining of the cervix.

They initially did two cryogenic freezes in the area in 2011, which did not stop the cell growth. She also had a more radical procedure, punch biopsy, to remove all cancerous cells surrounding the opening of the cervix. A follow up Pap in April 2011 was noted as "satisfactory" but she still tested positive for HPV.

She decided to start the silver sol gel protocol on May 15th, 2011. She also added the antioxidants and pH balancing foods.

On July 8th 2011 she tested HPV free and Pap test is clear of any atypical cells. She called in February of 2012 to give news of a normal Pap and HPV free test again. She said she is "ecstatic" about her results.

**Wendy R. 30**

Wendy came in for consultation on November 4th 2013. She is married and has one son, who just turned 2 years old. Prior to her son's 2nd birthday she had a Dilatation and Curettage (D&C) for abnormal bleeding. She also tested with an abnormal Pap noted as 'Severe Dysplasia CIN III or carcinoma in situ'. This is where the entire layer of epithelium is composed of abnormal cells. She is also HPV positive. Her OB/GYN had done a tissue biopsy from the D&C. She was diagnosed with cervical cancer. She had no symptoms, discharge, bleeding, or pain.

Her biggest fear at this time is financial. She worries about the cost of ongoing treatments or progression of cervical cancer.

Due to her history, she opted to do all the options, in addition to silver sol gel protocol. She did the silver sol for a week but used it with any intercourse and during menstruation as well. She focused on alkaline foods and leaner proteins as well as supplements.

December 16th 2013 she had a follow up Pap test which was CIN I. HPV negative.

In June of 2014 her Pap was negative and HPV negative. She continues to this day on a more alkaline diet, vitamin D3 supplementation, and uses silver sol gel frequently as a preventative.

**Elizabeth M. 41**

Client came in for a consultation on July 29th 2014. She gave a history of abnormal Pap Class II with hyperplasia of cervix and inflammation. She had tested positive for HPV. She was married twice and has three children from first husband with one spontaneous abortion. Her current concern was the routine Pap noted above. She admitted to multiple partners in adolescence. She gave an account of a rape when she was sixteen, non-consensual, at party she attended with underage drinking. This resulted in an unwanted pregnancy which was voluntarily aborted. She had a history of uterine bleeding prior to first child which BCP pills did not correct. She stated that the first pregnancy seemed to correct the abnormal bleeding disorder going forward but up until a year ago, she noticed abnormal bleeding happening again. So she went in for an exam with her OB/GYN and resultant Pap/HPV was positive.

She agreed to the silver sol gel protocol. In the course of consultation, emotions from her youth kept surfacing, so five flower therapy was suggested as an option, along with supplements of Vitamin D3, and antioxidants. She came back in for follow up consultation one week later on her own.

She stated in this visit that she was having a lot of flash backs to the rape event as a teen. She was instructed to use the flower therapy every 15 minutes under the tongue until this subtly subsided, which it did by the next day. I asked her to journal her thoughts and feelings about this. Her comments "I feel this rape has haunted my uterus for life". She felt she had a huge anger and fear issue which now seemed to release with the aid of flower therapy. Her comments and instincts are now to forgive her attackers.

She was instructed to do a follow up HPV test. This was negative on August 13th 2014. Pap was Class I and now considered "insignificant". She has continued with the supplements and feels "more energetic and safe". She felt lucky to have found such a powerful natural tool as silver sol gel and commented "why doesn't everyone know about this?"

**Theresa V. 44**

Inflammation is a common find on Pap tests in general. Theresa came to our office on September 8th 2014 by referral of her friend, who had success with the silver sol gel protocol in the past (not one of the 18, as she was outside the study time line). Theresa's routine Pap done a month ago was noted as LGSIL (low grade squamous intraepithelial lesions) –cell changes caused by HPV, also called CIN I mild dysplasia caused by HPV. A high degree of inflammation was also noted on the test results. She had not had an abnormal Pap test in the past prior to this one. She had been on a trip six months ago to Spain where she met someone, who she had a sexual encounter with, and had unprotected sex. She is divorcee as of two years ago. She said this encounter was not like anything she has ever done in the past and considers herself very conservative.

The reason she had this Pap was a "gut feeling" she had about this encounter. No symptoms were present, but she felt compelled to have a Pap test for peace of mind. Her physician instructed her to return in six months and have a follow up Pap.

She agreed to the silver sol gel protocol. Her diet was what she considers "Mediterranean" and is considered very healthy, per her lab blood work, and is on no medications. She did use antioxidant supplements along with the silver sol gel.

Her follow up Pap on November 5th 2014 was negative, well before her six months re-test. She stated her doctor remarked that "I told you it would clear up on its own. HPV is very common but nothing to be concerned about". Theresa strongly disagrees and is thankful for a natural holistic approach such as this versus just waiting.

**Yolinda V. 33**

Yolinda came to our office from Ontario Canada February 3rd 2013. She visits Wisconsin in the winter and heard about the silver sol protocol from another client. She has one child and runs a fly out fishing post. Her history included smoking but quit two months ago. No medications or surgeries.

She had been experiencing a foul odor vaginally. She has current complaints of vaginal itching and genital warts. She had a Pap test in January which was CIN II with moderate dysplasia and HPV positive, which this was recommended due to her history of genital warts. She indicated "a lot of white creamy discharge vaginally, that is yeasty". Her diet is very high carbohydrate laden and high protein. She eats very limited vegetables or fruits.

She agreed to the silver sol gel protocol and a pH balancing diet. She wishes to lose weight as well. She also agreed to the antioxidant supplements. We discussed her to continue on the pH balancing alkaline diet, lowering carbohydrate intake, and continuing on antioxidants. Especially due to her winter months in Canada and poor diet availability living in the far reaches of northern Ontario. She has limited access to fruits and vegetables.

She was instructed to follow up by phone and have a Pap re-test upon returning to Canada. On March 31st 2013 she called to report her Pap as normal. Her symptoms were extremely diminished, no odor but a small amount of discharge continues. She remarked the diet changes have been "hell for her". But she did report losing 9 pounds. Her itching is gone. The genital warts are still there. She asked if it is ok to continue the silver sol gel topically and internally (vaginal) as she felt it was a miracle. We discussed that it is a non-toxic substance and considered a class I medical device.

Yolinda called July 16th 2013. All her symptoms have subsided although her warts are only fifty percent gone. She has lost 15 pounds and kept it off. She also has a garden now and focuses heavily on alkaline fruits, vegetables, and whole grains.

She returned to our office February 19th 2014. I did not recognize her. She had lost 23 pounds and is currently pregnant. She reported no symptoms and her Pap follow up In January 2014 was negative. She continues using silver sol gel for prevention with intercourse. Her warts are now completely gone.

**Diane R. 47**

Diane gave a history on her consult of August 19th 2013 of an abnormal Pap smear and high-risk HPV infection when she was 35. At that time she had a LEEP Cone biopsy for "CIN II"or moderate dysplasia. She had other slightly abnormal Pap smears prior until she was 40. Recently, her last Pap test showed CIN I mild dysplasia and HPV positive. She is not married, but has been in long-term relationships and has mostly used condoms. She noted painful intercourse at times.

She started the silver sol gel protocol for a week. She opted to do nothing else.

She had a repeat Pap and HPV test in September of 2013 which was negative. She continues to use the gel for foreplay and intercourse as a preventative.

She has been HPV negative for two years now and stated she is very thankful there is a natural gel like this she can rely on, and wanted to know why her "physician didn't recommend this?"

**Nancy T. 38**

Nancy is a professional singer who is single and came to our office on April 16th 2014. She had been experiencing recent spotting in between her menstrual periods. She had never had a Pap test prior to this spotting. Her physician advised a Pap test and a HPV test per office guidelines and her current age. The test was positive for HPV and noted as ASCUS (Atypical squamous cells of undetermined significance). She was advised to return in one year.

Nancy is very concerned about cervical cancer and had lost a friend to cancer. She wanted to be more proactive than wait for a follow up Pap a year from now.

She agreed to do the silver sol gel protocol. She also added Vitamin D3 supplements of 2,000 IU/d per day. She also was taking 200mg of Eleuthro (ginseng) per day prior to admission into the protocol. It was agreed she could continue as this is part of the options but maybe up it to 500mg. She advised her doctor she was doing this and he advised that it "wasn't necessary, but I will monitor you if you wish. We would be happy to do a follow up Pap if you feel it is necessary so soon, but it may be out of pocket". Nancy felt that her doctor was already doing that, monitoring. Her comment was "This is my body, my money, and I am not going to do nothing".

She had a repeat Pap/HPV test done May 12th 2014 that was negative.

**Samantha E. 34**

She presented with an abnormal Pap and positive HPV test on October 21st of 2013. The Pap was classified as CIN I mild dysplasia caused by HPV taken on October 8th. She is married with four children and is a non-smoker.

She has had no symptoms to report, prior to this routine Pap test she had done on October 8th. She had two Pap tests previously done before October 8th, both without an HPV test. Her Pap test one year ago however, did show inflammation, but it was considered insignificant. She was advised to do a follow up Pap test two years later.

Samantha wanted to be included in the silver sol gel protocol as she heard about it from a friend who also participated in this study. She used only the silver sol gel for a week as outlined in the checklist.

She called November 18th 2013 to report all tests were "clear" or negative. She commented she "had to convince her practitioner to retest at her own cost, because insurance would not cover it. But her doctor was very interested in the study outcome results. Her doctor wants to see if this type of therapy could work, even though she most likely could not recommend it". Because she went on to say "her doctor could not prescribe it anyway, as it is considered over the counter treatment for HPV. But her doctor would be happy to refer people to the study if it works".

In Samantha's words "it obviously does work, did you see my Pap results?" Samantha feels this is a low cost alternative to just "waiting and seeing" if it HPV will clear on its own. "Why would anyone want to let a virus continue to invade their tissue and not be diligent about it? Cancer of the cervix is every woman's concern. I don't think they have a cure for it. Wait for what, surgery? I hope this becomes an option someday for all women". She is very vocal about it, as I have overheard her in natural health talks she attends that I give, to all who listen.

**Grace A. 36**

She entered our office on October 7th 2014. She had been in for a routine pap smear 2 years ago after her second son was born and was shocked to be diagnosed with pre-cancerous cells and tested HPV positive. She had previously considered vaccination for HPV with Gardasil (admitted to one dose). She was not sexually active as a teenager, she voiced she did not have multiple partners, and there was no history of cancer in her family. She spent about a month in shock after the routine Pap, she expressed this during consult. She was even admitted for counseling due to the shock of it. She was told "to complete your family and have your cervix removed".

She commented that her doctor did not have a good bedside manner. She decided to undergo the silver sol gel protocol with follow up tests before surgery. She wanted to exhaust any option before surgery. She agreed silver sol gel protocol, flower therapy, antioxidant supplements, and was advised to schedule some follow up Pap smears. To help show results of this therapy she was to have one Pap test done for next month. Her physician disagreed, but she did convince her to do this as a measure of the silver sol gel protocol, even though it was at her own expense.

Her Pap in November was noted to have no precancerous cells at all. She felt like "she was living a dream". She asked her follow up physician if the cancer "might have gone into remission". He said "no, it must not have ever been there to begin with". She told us that she is in "shock of a good kind, all over again, but it's a good thing".

She cancelled the December Pap test, her doctor agrees, but did call us to say she will get another one in 2015. Just to make sure. She is willing to continue the protocol as she said "I do not want to have my cervix removed anytime soon".

**Kathy R. 41**

Kathy came in for a consult on August 16th 2014.

Her history included multiple abnormal Pap tests over the years prior to 2010. She had cryosurgery back in 2010 because of those tests, with two subsequent Pap tests (2011 & 2012) which were considered negative.

In January of 2013, she had some pain in the pelvic region and spotting. She insisted on a Pap test and her Pap test came back CIN II. Hysterectomy was advised due to the history. She declined and was put on a follow up. Her most recent Pap in July of 2014 showed Severe Dysplasia CIN III or carcinoma in situ. She had been positive for HPV in the past.

Kathy wishes to do something naturally and not have a hysterectomy if she can avoid it. She is in consult with her OB/GYN. She has agreed to try the silver sol gel protocol and all options are to be implemented. Her doctor has agreed to monitor this but tests may not be covered by insurance and Kathy agreed. Her doctor has given her three months to change this or total Hysterectomy is practical.

Kathy's history is she is a non-smoker. She is currently married with one child. She admits to being promiscuous in college with multiple sexual partners. She did use BCP's in her youth. Currently on blood pressure medication only.

She followed all options on the checklist in addition to the one week silver sol gel protocol. Due to the carcinoma in situ it was advised she continue silver sol gel more often but first get a follow up Pap after the one week. She did and on August 26th her repeat Pap had come back CIN II. Her doctor was encouraged and shocked. HPV was negative.

Kathy continued the silver sol gel for three months using one to two times a week vaginally with tampon inserts, pH diet, and all supplements. She only took flower therapy the first week and felt no need to continue it as she noticed little effect.

On November 17th her follow up Pap was completely clear. Kathy is very pleased. She continues to take antioxidants, vitamin D3, and uses silver sol gel with her menstrual cycles as prevention. Kathy and her doctor were both stunned by this turn of events. Her physician refers positive HPV patients to this clinic as of now.

# Chapter 16:
# CONCLUSION

There seems to be no cure for HPV infection by traditional medicine today, only detection and treatment after detection.

Current recommended practices which include preventative hygiene and the use of debatable vaccinations (based on the Merck manual and CDC), are not stemming the tide of cervical cancer. As discussed, vaccines themselves seem to have very serious side effects with the potential to cause even more harm than good. This may tend to "fly in the face" of the Hippocratic Oath of "first, does no harm". Based on the case studies, a quantum and holistic approach using aqua sol silver technology is a viable and statistically sound integrated approach to HPV infection, also with preventative hygiene.

The history of silver in medicine and the advancement of silver into a silver sol are very well documented here. It has been demonstrated here that silver sol gel can block HPV viral entry and its effects. As the case studies prove, silver sol gel prohibits the HPV from binding to the surface of cells, and the virus is rendered ineffective. Silver sol gel also has immune assisting benefits by inhibiting bacteria (even Candida) which result in secondary infections.

It was also shown that silver sol has a documented synergy with antibiotics, making it a truly integrated product for the future of all of medicine. Silver sol gel can be used preventively or for treatment. It has been researched to be safe and effective with no side effects. If anything, it is full of side benefits. As evidence of the 18 case studies here, shown not in just theory, but in actual practice.

There are multiple reasons why an infection like HPV starts and flourishes in the first place. The documentation of these 18 female volunteers, along with the monitoring of their conventional physicians, has demonstrated a 100% recovery using the silver sol gel and options protocol.

The number of volunteers in this protocol maybe too small to draw 100% effectiveness conclusion to silver sol gel for every HPV infection, but has definitely shown a safe and noninvasive way to treat HPV infection in at least these 18 women. No one treatment is ever 100 percent effective for 100 percent of the people using it. But in this small case sampling, it did.

In the case of most people who use an alternative approach, they tend to use it much later on in a health challenge, only after conventional treatments have failed. As a general rule here the sooner you apply the silver sol protocol, after an abnormal Pap or positive HPV test is confirmed, the better. Chances of recovery (logic serves) are even more enhanced if used before the HPV virus has a chance to destroy any cellular DNA to begin with.

Conventional allopathic treatment really has no answer to this ongoing worldwide disease at this time. That doesn't mean there are not any other options, just not conventional ones. Further research on this type of non-toxic approach could further improve it and allow it to be combined with conventional treatments. Integration with this protocol can produce even more optimal results than just vaccination research or Pap smear monitoring alone.

Public opinion is changing about alternative care. Vital energy technology has been around for a long time. It is inexpensive by comparison to allopathic methods. Maybe even the insurance industry, if they could stand behind this less costly type of care, might actually stand to save money because of a less costly approach! Interesting to note, there are 1.5 million people who work in the health insurance industry, while barely half as many doctors provide the actual care. Health care is America's single largest industry. It is one of the average American's largest expenses (85). Silver sol has tremendous value of a less costly and integrated approach to HPV and cervical cancer.

In some of the case studies, a few physicians who were following the volunteers made comments like "I don't know what this is, but keep doing it". It is a fact that physicians can't prescribe this type of protocol anyway. But experts like Dr. Cynthia Eaton, Dr. Gordon Pedersen, Dr. Friedman, Paul Carlton Jr., just to name a few, would argue in favor of it.

Let's keep in mind every person is unique. Also are their conditions. But this outcome, based on the 18 case studies, does deserve attention. It is encouraged by this author that others try to duplicate this protocol for similar results in other patients. Large scale formal studies on silver sol gel won't be done by pharmaceutical companies or laboratories, they don't stand to profit.

This compilation has proven that not all options have been exhausted in the care and management of HPV infection. It has also shown there is a great deal of efficacy of treatment with silver sol gel, in conjunction with a holistic approach. It demonstrated a low level of difficulty in administration. That it is noninvasive, cost effective, and requires very little supervision. It was not expected to see 100% effectiveness in these 18 participants, but very welcome.

I hope this opens more eyes and encourages traditional medical doctors or universities to continue to explore silver sol technology, not only HPV, but for other potential applications as well.

In the realm of microorganisms such as virus, quantum physics gives us a better understanding of where medicine needs to go in the future. Frequency modulation, magnetic disruption, and cellular communication are quantum holistic principles and advance the idea of pleomorphism. The scientific research shown here about silver technology has overwhelming evidence of its efficacy. Skeptical or not, the information proves we need to bring forward quantum understanding and quantum doctors for the advancement of medicine from what nature has to offer.

Although centered on silver sol technology in HPV in women (decreasing cervical cancer), we must employ all diagnosis as a more systemic condition of body, mind, and soul. As long as we continue to break down the human condition (and its limitless possibilities) into just pieces, parts, and symptoms, we are not in harmony with the universal nature of true healing. We call it 'practicing medicine'. The goal shouldn't be just to cure a disease or manage one, but provide healing tools and energy for the whole health of an individual. If done correctly, "cure" will happen anyway. The body's vital energy and consciousness is what heals us, it happens no other way.

As discussed, modern science and traditional medicine is still firmly focused on monomorphism. It continues on an attempt to destroy a mass, tumor, or pathogen, and if so, assumes it won the battle. There is little emphasis on biological terrain or morphogenetic fields. As this is ignored, dis-ease most likely will reappear later as some other condition (symptoms) begging us to change. Ignoring pleomorphism concepts for example, remains an unchecked predisposition and epigenetic in nature. The patient is then never truly cured.

The Yellow Emperor's Classic on Internal Medicine, 500 B.C. stated "The physician who teaches people to sustain their health is the superior physician. The physician who waits to treat people until after their health is lost is considered inferior. This is like waiting until one's family is starving to begin to plant seed's in the garden."

Quantum creativity helps form the future of medicine, a quantum medicine. It started with concepts of a quantum nature such as biological terrain and epigenetics. The evidence is in that quantum ideas like, using silver sol gel on a tampon does deter HPV infection.

I leave you with these phrases: "You don't catch a cold, you earn one" and "may you never know the disease you prevented". To look to the future of medicine, rediscover the past. Go ahead be Quantum!

# References

A strong mention goes out here: Much of what has advanced from colloidal silver to silver aqua sol (structured silver/gold sol), has to be attributed to Dr. Gordon Pederson, N.D., Ph.D., in Toxicology. M.S. – Cardiac Rehabilitation and Wellness. Director of the Institute of Alternative Medicine. Chair - U.S. Pharmacopoeia Review Board Natural Products Committee. Board Certified Anti-Aging and Regenerative Medicine. He performed his cardiology internship at LDS Hospital under direct supervision of Jonas Salk (polio vaccine).

Some of this research would not have been possible without his pioneering efforts and permission. Thank you to Dr. Gordon Pederson and for the use of his pictures. But more importantly "thank you" Gordon for your untiring dedication to helping find quantum solutions to help heal God's children.

(1) www.cdc.gov/nchs/data/dvs/lead1900_98.pdf

(2) JAMA June 14, 2000 – Vol. 283, No. 22, pg. 2977 Are Increasing 5-Year Survival Rates Evidence of Success against Cancer?

(3) http://cid.oxfordjournals.org/content/32/4/e69.full

(4) The Merck manual of Diagnosis & Therapy. Nineteenth edition pg. 2576, 2578, 2579, 2580.

(5) http://en.wikipedia.org/wiki/Human_papillomavirus

(6) Silver Solutions. Special Report: Women's Health. Dr. Cynthia Eaton, Dr. Gordon Pederson DVD. 2009 Sound Concepts.

(7) http://biology.about.com/od/cellbiology/ss/normal-cells-cancer-cells.htm

(8) Digest Journal of Nanomaterials and Biostructures Vol. 9, No. 1, January - March 2014, p. 175 – 186. Application of Silver Nanoparticles in Viral Inhibition: A New Hope for Antivirals. N. Khandelwal, G. Kaur, N. Kumara, A. Tiwari

(9) 2012 Cervical Cancer Prevention, Dr. Patricia Yarberry Allen, gynecologic oncologist Monica Prasad, HPV, new guidelines on Pap smears.

(10) Kiviat, N.B., and L.A. Koutsky. 1993. Specific human papillomavirus types as the causal agents of most cervical intraepithelial neoplasia: implications for current views and treatment. J. Natl. Cancer Inst. 85:934-935.

(11) Vaccine (Merck) pg. 1176

(12) www.cdc.gov/vaccinesafety/Vaccines/HPV/jama.html

(13) Time magazine, February 9, 2015, The Vaccine Crisis

(14) www.theonc.org/author.asp?doc_id=265168

(15) http://www.scirp.org/journal/PaperInformation.aspx?PaperID=25840

(16) Pederson Gordon Ph.D. N.D., The Silver Solution to Women's Wellness. Second Edition 2011

(17) Pedersen Gordon Ph.D., N.D., FAPWCA, FAARM. A New Fighting Chance, Silver Solution. A Quantum Leap in Silver Technology: How molecular structuring safely destroys bacteria, viruses and yeast. Fourth Edition 2014

(18) Orrin Hatch. Letter to Hon. Tom Ridge Homeland Security, 2006.

(19) www.silverhealthinstitute.com

(20) Merck Index. 1999, Silver, 1:645.

(21) http://en.wikipedia.org/wiki/Argyria

(22) Nelson Labs, Brigham Young University. 2005.

(23) Pedersen, Gordon, Ph.D., N.D., Alkaline Structured Silver; Mechanisms of Action and the Nano-Electrocution of Disease Causing Pathogens

(24) DeSouza, A. D. Mehta., Current Science Investigation, 91(7), 2006. Bactericidal activity of combination of Silver-Water dispersion with 19 antibiotics against seven microbial strains.

(25) Pedersen G, Hegde B M, The Indian Practitioner Sept. 2010, Vol. 63, No. 9, Silver Sol Completely Removes Malaria Parasites from the Blood of Human Subjects Infected with Malaria in an Average of 5 days: A Review of Four Randomized, Multi-Centered, Clinical Studies Performed in Africa.

(26) Hafkine, A., 2003. ASAP antiviral activity in Hepatitis B; DNA Polymerase Inhibition, Reverse Transcriptase Inhibition. Hafkine Institute for Training, Research, and Testing.

(27) http://www.hydrosolinfo.com/articles/silver-2004-12-22.php

(28) Ghana Food and Drug Board New drug approval, 2007

(29) Journal of nanobiotechnology; 3:6 (2005). J. L. BJL Elechiguerra, J. R. Morones, A. Camacho-Bragado, X. Gao, H. H. Lara, M. J. Yacaman

(30) Journal of Nanobiotechnology.8, 1 (2010). H. H. A-NNV Lara, L. Ixtepan-Turrent, C. Rodriguez-Padilla

(31) Journal of Nanobiotechnology.8:15 (2010). H. H. I-TL Lara, E. N. Garza-Trevino, C. Rodriguez-Padilla

(32) Chemical Communications. (40):5059 (2005). R. W. CR Sun, N. P. Chung, C. M. Ho, C. L. Lin, C. M. Che.

(33) Antiviral Therapy. 13(2):253 (2008). L. SRW Lu, R. Chen, C. K. Hui, C. M. Ho, J. M. Luk, G. K. Lau, C. M. Che.

(34) Antivir. Ther. 2008, 13:253–262. Lu L, Sun RW, Chen R, Hui CK, Ho CM, Luk JM, Lau GK, Che CM: Silver nanoparticles inhibit hepatitis B virus replication.

(35) Journal of Nanobiotechnology. 8, 19 (2010). J. L. MRC Speshock, L. K. Braydich-Stolle, A. M. Schrand, S. M. Hussain.

(36) I. SC Papp, K. Ludwig, M. Roskamp, C. Bottcher, S. Schlecht, A. Herrmann, R. Haag. Inhibition of influenza virus infection by multivalent sialic-acid-functionalized gold nanoparticles. Small; 6(24), 2900 (2010).

(37) Bioconjugate chemistry.20 (8), 1497 (2009). D. SS Baram-Pinto, N. Perkas, A. Gedanken, R. Sarid.

(38) Journal of Biomedical Nanotechnology. 4(2):149 (2008). SAK Sun Lova, Vig Komal, R. Pillai Shreekumar, R. Singh Shree

(39) Genetics and Molecular Research 13 (3): 7022-7028 (2014).

(40) Roy, R., Current Science Investigation, 2007. Ultradilute Ag-aquasols with extraordinary bactericidal properties: role of the system Ag-O-H2O.

(41) General P.K. Carlton MD. Letter to the Department of Homeland Security. 2007.

(42) Lyons, Barry - The Cancer Cure That Worked

(43) Institute for Antiviral Research. Silver Sol and H5N1 Influenza, 2005

(44) http://www.silverhealthinstitute.com/silver-viruses/

(45) Robinson, R., 2003. Bactericidal activity of ASAP Silver Solution on Yersinia Pestis, the etiological agent of plague. Department of Microbiology, Brigham Young University.

(46) Viridis Biopharma, 3:2004. Selective Inaction of ASAP on Probiotics

(47) Carr, H. Wlodowski, T. 1973. Dept. of Microbiology, College of Physicians and Surgeons, Columbia University, New York, New York. Antimicrobial Agents and Chemotherapy. 10:585-587

(48) EPA #D011

(49) http://www.silverhealthinstitute.com/rustum-roy-waters-structure-colloidal-silver-new-vectors/

(50) Pedersen, G., Moeller K., Journal of the Science of Healing Outcomes., (2009)., Silver Sol Improves Wound Healing: Case Studies in the use of Silver Sol in closing wounds (including MRSA) preventing infection, inflammation and activating stem cells.

(51) Pedersen, Gordon, Ph.D., N.D., Alkaline Structured Silver; Mechanisms of Action and the Nano-Electrocution of Disease Causing Pathogens

(52) Emoto Masaru, The Miracle of Water 2007, http://en.wikipedia.org/wiki/Hexagonal_water

(53) Khan, MS, Vishakanie, CD., Siddaramaiah, H. Curr Drug Metab. 2012 Oct; 13(8): 1119-22. Gold nanoparticles: a paradigm shift in biomedical applications

(54) Muhammad, N, Guo, Z., Curr Opin. Chem Biology. 2014 March 5:19c:153 Metal Based Anticancer Chemotherapeutic Agents

(55) Antimicrobial and barrier effects of silver against methicillin-resistant Staphylococcus aureus. Edwards-Jones V. Journal of Wound Care. 2006 Jul;15(7):285-90

(56) Zeller, J.L. et al. "JAMA patient page. MRSA infections." JAMA 2007 Oct. 17; 298(15): 1826

(57) Surgeons Scrub Test Protocol using Silver Aquasol 2005. www.silverhealthinstitute.com

(58) http://www.who.int/mediacentre/news/releases/2014/amr-report/en/

(59) Becker RO, Spadaro JA. J Bone & Joint Surgery. 1978;60;871

(60) Flick AB, Platte V. Clinical applications of electrical silver iontophoresis

(61) University of Cal Davis. Silver Sol and healthy intestinal flora. 2005

(62) Fox, C.J., Control of Pseudomonas Infection in Burns by Silver Sulfadiazine. Surg. Gynecol. Obstet. 128:1021-1026

(63) CBTRUS 1995-1999 Statistical Report: primary brain Tumors in the United States.

(64) Conclusions from the Children's Cancer group 921 randomized phase III study. J. Clinical Oncology 17:832-845, 1999

(65) Pierce, Tanya Harter M.A., MFCC, Outsmart your Cancer. Alternative Non-Toxic Treatments that Work. Pg. 119, 120.

(66) http://en.wikipedia.org/wiki/Vaginal_flora

(67) http://cid.oxfordjournals.org/content/32/4/e69.full

(68) Sugrue, Thomas., There is a River: Story of Edgar Cayce

(69) JAMA Measuring the Quality of Hospital-based Domestic Violence Programs (2002;287:177)

(70) Rajalakshmi, K., Epigenetics as a Solution in Autism: Control above Autism Genes 2015

(71) Jeffrey Smith - leading spokesperson on the health dangers of genetically modified organisms (GMOs) 2003 Seeds of Deception).

(72) (46.6) http://www.nature.com/ejhg/journal/v14/n2/full/5201567a.html

(73) Das M, Dixit S, Khanna SK. Food additives and contaminants. 2005

(74) J. Biological Chemistry 2011 Jul 22;286(29):25586-603

(75) http://ocra-oregon.org/foodsthatfightcancer.pdf

(76) http://vitalforcetechnology.energytoolsint.com/dr-yury-kronn

(77) Gerber, Richard M.D., Vibrational Medicine – New Choices for Healing Ourselves 1996

(78) Goswami, Amit Ph.D., Physics of the Soul 2013

(79) Nelson Laboratories March 3, 2009 USP 51 for 24ppm Silver Sol, Antimicrobial Preservative Effectiveness Test #459306

(80) Conners, Kevin D.C. FICA, ABAAHP Beating Chronic Lyme. April 2013

(81) Veugelers PJ. Ekwaru JP 2014, Vieth 199, Hathcock 2007, Ekwaru JP et al. 2014 www.purenorth.ca

(82) Simone, C.B., et al. Antioxidants and other nutrients do not interfere with Chemotherapy or Radiation therapy and can increase kill and survival, Part I. Alternative Therapies. 2007 Jan/Feb; 13 (1): 22-28. Part II, 2007 Mar/Apr; 13 (2): 40-47

(83) Diamond, W. John., M.D., W. Lee Cowden, M.D. and Burton Goldberg. An Alternative Medicine Definitive Guide to Cancer. Tiburon, California: Future Medicine Publishing, Inc. 1997, p. 617.

(84) Ritchason, Jack N.D., The Little Herb Encyclopedia. The Third Edition 1995

(85) Brill, Steven., Americas Bitter Pill 2015

44878621R00069

Made in the USA
San Bernardino, CA
25 January 2017